Surviving *the* FITNESS GAME

28 Day

Devotional Workout

Bridge-Logos

Alachua, Florida 32615 USA

Bridge-Logos

Alachua, FL 32615 USA

Surviving the Fitness Game
by JoAnna Ward

Printed in the United States of America.

Library of Congress Catalog Card Number: 2007942358
International Standard Book Number 978-0-88270-458-6

G616.316.N.m712.352100

Dedicated in loving memory to
my mother, Dorothy Vassell,
who transitioned into eternity
August 28, 2002

*"And we know that all things work together for good
to them that love God, to them who are the
called according to his purpose."*
Romans 8:28

CONTENTS

PART 1: PREPARATION FOR FITNESS

Introduction. 1
Prayer That Changes the Weight Loss Game. 6

Surviving the Mental Game: A New Mind 11

The Mind Game: Balance & Beauty in a Ball. 12
Mind Over Matters. 13
A Made-Up Mind: Prayer 15

Surviving the Spiritual Game: Spiritual Weightlifting 17
Spiritual "Heaviness" 17
Reality: A Spiritual Casting Call 18
Spiritual Restoration. 24
Spiritual Speech: Prayer 28

Surviving the Body Shaping Game: Master Building 31
A "Triangle" Building: Mind, Body, Soul. 31
Building Habits. 34
Blessing the Building: Prayer 38

Confessional Conclusion 41

PART 2:
"PEACES" OF THE PINEAPPLE

A 28-Day Devotional

Introduction 45
Pineapples in the Jungle 53
Discipline in a "Foreign Land" 55

"Peaces" of the Pineapple 59
Daily Disciplines 60
Understanding the Grid 64
Power Grid 66
Week 1: Fruit of Praise 69
Week 2: Fruit of the Spirit 93
Week 3: Fruit of Obedience 121
Week 4: Fruit of Sacrifice 143

Descriptions and Instructions for Core Exercises 175
Core 1: Cardio Exercises 175
Core 2: Leg Work Exercises 178
Core3: Arm Work Exercises 181
Core 4: Abdominal Work Exercises 184
Core 5: Ball Work Exercises 186

Acknowledgments 197

PART I

Preparation
for
FITNESS

Introduction

As we pass through life, our purpose is issued to us one moment at a time. Our time on the Earth is so special that we could not fast forward to even the next five minutes if we wanted to. We must take life as it comes. The better prepared we are to deal with life coming at us 110 miles per hour, the more success we will find along the way. We may continue to ignore it or water it down with quick-fix solutions, but weight loss, like all phases of life, takes time, preparation, and commitment.

Weight *gain* is a slow and gradual process. So is weight *loss*. In an attempt to lose weight, many people rush toward their aspirations and miss the essence of the experience. Perfected daily routines produce success and the accomplishment of daily goals. While this application may be applied to accomplishing weight loss goals, it may be tough, at first, because the body will resist going into the rarely visited territories of self-control and self-discipline. Many weight loss goal setters have attempted success only to end up in the territory of self-defeat. You, however, have no need to worry. You have the right plan in your hand. Give yourself just one more shot at getting your weight under control. More importantly, give God complete control through the power of His Holy Spirit. That's right!

This book is Holy Spirit-inspired and guided. Look forward to a new mind. Look forward to a new heart, both physical and spiritual. Look forward to a new body. Look beyond the past attempts of self-defeat and self-despair and allow self-discipline and the Most High God, the creator of Heaven and Earth, and the creator of you, to transform your entire being!

Destiny takes time and preparation. If you fail to prepare, you prepare to fail. Often, challenges and difficulties inadvertently transform us into the people God predestined us to be. For example, I was a track star in high school. Each year, I claimed the title of Best All-Around. My mother would often remind me that I had been running like the wind since I was two years old. She confirmed that I would run back and forth throughout the house for what seemed like hours. I had been preparing to become a runner long before I actually became recognized as one. God knew His plan for my life, and, without anyone's permission or foreknowledge, He began preparing me.

Likewise, I was prepared to be a contestant on CBS's "Survivor: Amazon." Long before there was a show created by Mark Burdett, I was a survivor. Long before the initial interview process, I was a survivor. Long before I was chosen as a member of the sweet sixteen finalist group, I was chosen by God to proclaim His praises. Long before I was a castaway in the game, I had overcome being a castoff in life. I am a survivor, but this design of my life runs deeper than just being a contestant on a reality TV show. The role of survivor in my destiny was cast long before my stay on the show and will continue until the moment I exit the stage of life. This role is best defined by a life overwhelmed with setbacks, challenges, obstacles, and big bad wolves. Yet, we can overcome them all by the blood of the lamb. I am a survivor, and I know that there is a survivor in you.

Before I devoted my life to God, I was devoted to my basketball scholarship that demanded good grades and a firm physical commitment. Four forty-five a.m. was the set time for morning practice. This time seemed overwhelmingly early for me. I would grow restless and anxious the night before for fear of oversleeping. I had no idea that God was preparing me for the forth watch, which is the darkest hour. He was preparing me to rise before daybreak, knowing that this training would prepare me for spiritual growth and development, and warfare. At the time, it just seemed hard and unnecessary to wake up so early in the morning. What was the point? Would it really make us play better basketball? Yes, we played better basketball, but, more importantly, this strenuous, well-organized training made us great and highly disciplined women.

Once I finally dedicated my life to Christ, it was almost like the Holy Spirit tapped into a spiritual storage pantry I had inside of me full of all those seemingly pointless experiences. The Holy Spirit began to pull me out of bed in the early morning hours for spiritual training and study with the same tenacity and consistency I had as a student athlete. Instead of studying the theories and practices of Abraham Maslow and the flawed Skinner box, I began to study and practice the Word of God. There was tremendous transformation and growth in my life.

Every morning, I woke with an excitement to worship, study, and fellowship with my heavenly Father. I would get up, get out, and run up and down and around the entire stadium. I would run just like I had done for the past twenty-five years, only this time it was for destiny. I would clear sections of the stadium in reverse order beginning at R and working my way to A. My body would be so physically challenged in completing the run that my mind and spirit would be given free reign to exercise, create, grow, and flow. As my body was distracted by the workout, my spirit engaged the power of the Holy Spirit,

3

and I would leave the stadium replenished with great revelation, insight, and truth.

One day, as I finished the nearly five-hundred steps elevated to over fifty feet in most sections, I heard the word of the Lord. "This is not about you, and you need to worship me. How many people do you think have the stamina to do this every day? This is not about you, and you need to worship me." I began saying "Hallelujah" at the top of my voice, and it rang throughout the stadium. Then it turned into a song of worship. "Hallelujah…Oh Glory…Hallelujah…Amen…"

I began to invite overweight people to join me, and they came. I would finish before them and began to worship the Lord in a mighty way. His Holy Spirit would fill that stadium. We were blessed. We would pray and God responded. Hundreds of pounds fell away. In a year's time, one lady lost over 103 pounds. We had no idea what God was really doing.

Against the admonishments and advice of some, I included this morning devotional as a vital aspect of my life on my audition tape for "Survivor: Amazon." Thank God that His foolishness is wiser than we are and His weakness is stronger than we are. The morning devotion coupled with before and after footage of the ladies caused my tape to stand out among the talent scouts. As a matter of fact, these two inclusions against "better" judgment were later noted as highlights of the tape. I clipped in the before and after video footage of The Jamison Sisters. I also included the four-word worship in the tape as well. This was the major ministry in the woman that I had become. God chose me to help these ladies who really loved Him and prayed for help and deliverance from their weight and overeating. The dramatic weight loss and change in countenance impressed the scouts so much that it landed me a spot on the show. Obviously, the praise and worship caught their attention as well.

I am convinced that God received the offering of worship that we sent up in that stadium each morning. As I lifted my voice in praise while under the enormous canopy of the Amazon rainforest amidst the animals, natives, other contestants, and the twenty-four-hour camera crew, God showed me just how seriously He takes devotion, dedication, and pure praise and worship. Praise is comely and it only offends the enemy of your soul. God took the same worship that was offered in that football stadium and allowed it to be heard around the world on an internationally-viewed television show each week. I call it "The World Wide Worship." I had no idea just how far it would go. I could feel every day that God would soon do something major, but to lift my eyes in the Amazon was beyond anything I could ever imagine. That experience was never conceived in my mind. Ironically, due to predestined preparation, maneuvering through the deadly jungle full of predators came easily to me. I took the Word of God that I could overcome the predators of surviving the game through the same Christ that strengthened me when the predators of life rose against me. There was a strategy for survival implemented in my life that was designed to help, encourage, and deliver others long before my eyes graced the white sands of the Amazon.

Now, by the grace of God, I present this strategic plan to you. God has a master plan for your life, and you have an obligation to position yourself to acquire the inheritance of your God-given destiny. This book provides fundamental steps in getting prepared to live an optimal life. Christ has come that we might have an abundant life. Walking in the abundant life begins with mental, spiritual, and physical preparation, and lots of self-discipline.

Prayer that Changes the Weight Loss Game

Preparing a Prayer Time

Please set aside a quiet time and place to come into agreement with me and every other reader of this book for prayer. You should say this prayer as often as the Holy Spirit leads you. You should meditate on its manifestation by faith. If every reader is constantly in one accord, praying the same prayer, to the same God, in the matchless name of Jesus Christ, I not only believe, but know, that our lives can and will be changed. See James 5:16. With all of the information, fitness challenges, recommendations, and suggestions to find solutions to health-related epidemics, the research, study, and grants, exercise equipment inventions, coupled with begging and pleading with people to get active and eat right, and even the scare tactics emphasizing sickness and death, I have firmly decided that only unified prayer can break a stronghold of this magnitude.

This problem is so big and profound that it has an imprisoning power over an entire nation. Nothing is too hard, big, or profound for God. He has promised that when we really cry out to Him in repentance and need that He will hear us and heal our land. "If my people, which are called by my name, shall *humble* themselves, and pray, and seek my face, and turn from their wicked ways; then will I hear from heaven, and will forgive their sin, and will HEAL their Land" (2 Chronicles 7:14, emphasis mine).

I know that our land is in need of a spiritual and physical healing from the Most High God, El-Elyon, through His Son, Jesus Christ. We do not need another prescription drug, another fad diet, or more quick-fix surgery. We must be healed. We must be delivered.

A Survivor's Prayer

Let's turn to Our Father in agreement and in prayer in the name of Jesus Christ:

Abba Father, we come together before you in one accord, agreeing with each other, believing and trusting in your faithfulness to respond to the effective and fervent prayers of the righteous. To begin, Father, we ask your forgiveness for not being faithful stewards over the bodies and health you have blessed us with. Forgive us for taking for granted our health and for treating our bodies harshly. Forgive us for not exercising self-control in our eating and self-discipline in keeping our bodies fine-tuned and in top condition.

Father God, we bless your Holy name for you are worthy, righteous, powerful and mighty. You are loving, kind, merciful, compassionate, gentle, and all-knowing. We thank you for a time such as this, and we thank you for our Lord and Savior Jesus Christ, for it is through our belief in His resurrection power that we know you hear us and answer us. It is through the resurrection power of Jesus Christ that we have authority over every stronghold in our lives. We ask you to put us in remembrance of stirring that authority daily and exercising it over our mouths, bellies, and everyday food choices. Lord, we thank you for willpower, and we praise you for the power of the Holy Spirit.

Thank you, Lord Jesus, for your obedience has allowed us to come boldly before the throne of grace, obtain mercy, and find help in our time of need. We need you, Father, individually, collectively, as a family, and as a nation. Father God, we need healing of a Divine kind. We need a touch from you, Oh Lord; we need a delivering touch from you. We bring our lives, our families, our community, and our home under the submission of your Holy Spirit to tear down the strongholds of storing excess fats and poor eating habits and remove the yoke of inactivity and laziness from our lives in the name of Jesus Christ.

Father God, help us to study, remember, and retain your word, as we shall not live by bread alone. Your Word, oh Lord, is a lamp unto our feet, leading and guiding and instructing us in the paths of righteousness for your namesake. We can do all things through Christ who strengthens us. Bless us to do these things without doubt, fear, or wavering, because you, oh Lord, have not given us a spirit of fear, but of love, and of power, and of a sound and disciplined mind.

Teach us, Father, through your Holy Spirit that leads us into all truth, to pray for wisdom when shopping for food. Give us wisdom and love in meal preparation. Grant us the strength to exercise portion control over all of our meals. Father God, give us knowledge and selectivity about where and how often to dine outside of our homes. Stir up the spirits of diligence and youthfulness in us to become more active with our children and spouses even through attending weekly worship services.

Fill us, Father God, with a peace that surpasses all understanding and an unspeakable joy at all times. Once again, Lord Jesus, bless our households, our marriages, our immediate, extended and church families, and our communities. Bless our nation. Holy Spirit, we invite you to dwell among us, take residence with us, and we give you permission and power of attorney over our lives to evict every spirit that is not like you or sent from the Father above. Remove any thing or person in our lives that opposes the destiny you alone, God, have outlined for us. If anything we do or say offends your Holy Spirit, please forgive us.

We submit and surrender our bodies to you as living, breathing sacrifices. Make us Holy and complete as you are Holy and complete. We are your masterpieces, not created apart from your very own image, but made in your likeness. Use our gifts and talents, and bind them together to strengthen the entire body of Christ. Be glorified not only when you complete this work in us, but, while you are doing this work in us, stir up a spirit of praise and an attitude of gratitude. For you are worthy to be praised.

Let everything that has breath, or breathes with the breath of life given to Adam, praise the Lord. Hallelujah! Oh Glory! Hallelujah! Amen!

Surviving the Mental Game:
A New Mind

"You will guard him and keep him in perfect and constant peace whose mind [both its inclination and character] is stayed on You, because he commits himself to You, leans on You, and hopes confidently in You" Isaiah 26:3 (AMPL).

The mind, second only to the heart, has the greatest influence over the body. Your brain is the control tower manipulated by your mind. Most of the warfare you experience at home, in your career, relationships, finances, and even with your weight or eating habits, originates in the mind. The emotional battlefield is established on the softened or hardened ground of the mind. Paul prayed for the mind of Christ. Christ walked with a set, perfect, sound. and made-up mind. Paul and Timotheus recognized divine power in the walk and life of Christ. They understood that in order to see deliverance and transformation in the Church at Philippi, the believers were going to need the mind of Christ (See Philippians 2:5). The effectiveness that Paul displayed without wavering in his faith indicates that this was not only part of his teaching, but his personal daily prayer. This is an empowering command that, when confessed over your life as a part of your daily devotion, gives you focus and clarity.

The Mind Game: Beauty & Balance in a Ball

As a college basketball player I remember our coach screaming, "Mind over matter, mind over matter, girls!" I later learned that was a common affirmation used in several branches of the United States military. To think: Our coach used military reinforcement quotes and drills just to win a few college basketballs games. OK, it was for those championships that only we care about now.

Our women's basketball team at South Carolina State University was not the most skilled team in the conference, and we did not have the top resources or facilities. While our team lacked top recruits and superstar players, we were laden with ladies who needed an education, loved the game, and had lots of heart. We had a coach who understood mental focus, discipline, and the game itself. Each fall, we would freelance scrimmage guys from the men's basketball team, the football team, and innocent bystanders who wanted to test their skill set against these well-disciplined, synchronized, intelligent, athletic, beautiful "girl" basketball players with so much game. While these guys could run faster, jump higher, and shoot farther than us, we were basketball players, not just a bunch of girls going through the motions of playing pick-up. We were college recruits hired to learn the game of basketball, while still being ladies, and win. We knew court awareness, balance, rhythm, timing and how to immediately identify the weaknesses of our opponents. This meant we missed very few opportunities to score on and off the court. We would win just about every time.

Our losses on the court were few and came within a point or two. These anomalies would only occur due to what our coach referred to as a "lack of mental focus" before dismissing us in sheer disappointment from his gym. His disappointment would only be pacified if a team really was better than we were. Losing focus, taking bad shots, missing lay-ups, playing half-hearted defense, or simply making a series of bad decisions, were not acceptable mishaps on his court. These mishaps were considered unacceptable for the scrappy survivors of the Lady Bulldogs and were just cause for us to get put out of the gym and into the dog house.

Although these were just past time pick-up games for the others, this was preparation for us. This really hurt because we loved the game, we wanted to win, and when we lost, we knew why. Being a champion was a 24-hours-a-day, 7-days-a-week, year-to-year mindset. In Bulldog Country, the mentality was not that of *Will we win tonight?*, but *How many points will we win by?* and *Can we bust the clock?* "Busting the clock" occurs when a team scores over a hundred points and the ticker is set back to zero. We went on to win several Mid-Eastern Athletic Conference and regular season and tournament championships.

Mind Over Matters

Hearing the words "Mind over matter, mind over matter" all of those years only made me work harder and keep going. It was not until I was an adult, teaching and inspiring others, that I realized what those words really meant. Most of my teammates and others still do not get the revelation of the military quote past a basic understanding to keep going, work harder, and that a stiff penalty awaits anyone slacking off.

Simply put: If you don't mind, it won't matter. My experiences have further taught me that this pendulum swings both ways. If you are content to die early, be obese, seriously ill or at high risk for illness, lonely, and insecure, then none of this will matter. On the other hand, if you don't mind sacrifices of being uncomfortable for about an hour or less, taking time out of your sleep or busy schedule to lend to fitness, or choosing to eat what is good for you over what is good to you, then it won't matter either. The sacrifice is then worth its weight in gold. Do you mind working hard for what you want? Not for a car or house or spouse, but for the health that you want and the body to go with it? Are you ready to change your mind?

Matters that Challenge the Mind

Every New Year's Eve, our willing spirits embrace the concept of a new and much-needed lifestyle change that usually includes adding exercise and losing some weight. We really believe that the new year sparks a new chance to really "do the doggone thing." The truth of the matter is that this opportunity awaits you at any time of the year, month, week, or day. Of course there are other occasions when people become hard pressed for an instant physical makeover, such as an upcoming cruise or vacation, a wedding, large gatherings, or just about any major "all eyes on me" event.

These are times and places of significance and remembrance, and you really want to look your best. There will be plenty of pictures, and most people want their photographed memories to be pleasant. But you cannot let them see you like this: thirty pounds overweight, more or less; that's not even you. You cannot have "them," whoever they are, talk and whisper behind your back. The fact that only people of low character and integrity would waste time on negatively discussing the struggles of another person does not faze you. The fact that your spouse and friends reassure you that no one is tracking your weight or thinking about it, gives you no consolation. The battle about how you look rages within your own mind. So you sit this one out and that one out and the next one out. Before your family and friends see you again, you have gained another thirty pounds, and you have grown depressed and borderline introverted. So, what happens to your plans to get fit? Where did that motivation go that you had at some point when you considered yourself serious about your fitness fate? What happened to the New Year's resolutions? Ninety-percent of all fitness goals go unmet because there is no preparation, no plan, no accountability, and the spirit and body were challenged without adequate mental preparation.

A Made-Up Mind: Prayer

You have to decide that your mind is what it is because you have allowed it to become what it is. You are the only person who can take control of where you are right now. You have an option. You have a choice. You can decide. If you are only "tired" of having excessive abdominal fat and being overweight, as soon as that temporary feeling of dissatisfaction and unhappiness fades, you will again grow complacent. You have to be fed up! You must be through with dealing with the habits that got you here in the first place. Once you have a full command of the mind over matter principle, then you will own the mental prowess to master your mouth, spirit, and body.

Prayer for My Mind

Father God, I ask that you continue to let the mind that was in Christ be in me also and that it would affect all aspects of my life. Holy Spirit, please take complete control

15

and embrace the weak parts of my will. I acknowledge that I cannot do this all by myself, but I can do all things through Christ who strengthens me. Christ Jesus, strengthen my mind and prepare me for this new lifestyle. Grant me mental temperance and self-control through the constant study of your Word. Lord, remind me to put the helmet of salvation over my mind daily so that my choices are guarded and my thoughts are sound. Holy Spirit, you are welcome to come in and be the new operator of the command center of my mind.

Father, I pray for the convicting power of the Holy Spirit to come upon me with any and every attempt I make to defile or corrupt your holy temple, my body. Help me to be a faithful steward over my mind and fill it with your Word and other forms of encouragement. Father God, help me to stay focused on your promises and the plans and goals that I am establishing for a better life. Father, I know that it is not by power, nor by might, but by your Holy Spirit, that I have victory in each situation, circumstance, and in all warfare that arises on the battlefield of my mind.

Bless this mind, Oh God, with your Godly wisdom, knowledge, and understanding that I might rule and subdue my own body according to your will and intentions for my life. Hallelujah! Oh Glory! Hallelujah! Amen!

Surviving the Spiritual Game: Spiritual Weightlifting

"The strong spirit of a man sustains him in bodily pain or trouble, but a weak and broken spirit who can raise up or bear?" Proverbs 18:14 (AMPL)

Spiritual "Heaviness"

Most of the ability to stay firmly focused on a fitness regimen is highly associated with strong mental focus and lightness of spirit. However, heaviness of spirit and mind can manifest within the body in the form of excessive weight gain. The weight gain is an outward manifestation of things going on in the minds and souls of people.

I have discovered through many counseling and consultation sessions that the onset of weight gain, obesity, or overeating is often derived from some sort of emotionally traumatic experience. Most people overeat to comfort themselves or because they are bored, hurt, or lonely. Some overeaters and under-exercisers have been rejected or misunderstood. I could go on and on as to the many reasons why people indulge in sedentary lifestyles perpetuated by overeating.

"A wounded spirit who can bear?"

The average physical weight gain of great proportions is correlated with a broken spirit. Yet spiritual brokenness is *not* manifested only in physical weight gain. I have ministered to women, men, and children who faired well on the scale, but they were morbidly obese in the spirit by 350 or more pounds! Spiritual heaviness is some of deadliest and most difficult weight to lose. However, exchanging the garment of heaviness for a garment of praise is sure to produce eternal joy while producing a high quality of earthly life.

Reality: A Spiritual Casting Call

Prior to a separation from my then-husband that led to a traumatic divorce, I only had associated my spirit with the afterlife and things associated with eternity. Until it was squeezed and ultimately crushed, I barely knew that it was that little thing that carried subliminal bitterness, anger, and an absence of forgiveness. I was totally oblivious. God knew over a decade ago that I would be writing this book and that you would need to read this testimony at this season in your life.

I had married my college sweetheart. He was a football player. I was a basketball player. We were a match made in Heaven, literally. I am not kidding. I had knowledge of my mother's God and her system of attending church, but no spiritual foundation of my own. I thank God for a praying mother, Dorothy Vassell, whose prayers covered and kept me from hundreds of miles away and whose personal walk taught me of the Lord Jesus Christ. It is vital that we teach our children of the Lord so that, when they are old, they will have a foundation to return to and on which to build their own relationship with Christ. Macey and I had both been taught better, and we knew that premarital sex was against God's laws, but, because we did not mind, it did not matter. Also, we would both learn the very lesson as to why God consistently warns about fornication in His Word. From the front of the Bible to the back, fornication is frowned upon and chastised. The law about fornication was for our own good. God is already good. My junior year in college, during an MEAC Championship Tournament, Macey drove many hours to cheer us on to a stellar victory and assist me in conceiving our only child together, Dontre.

Spiritual Conception

I realized about a month later that I was pregnant, and I could not afford to be. I was bent on having an abortion. My spirit was still asleep in my mind, obviously, because I did not think twice about it. It was the only option, right? Macey opposed me the entire time, but I was a force to be reckoned with. I was a prime athlete with a mind over matter concept that could not be shaken. I could care less about Macey's feelings and never asked God anything because He was not in it when it started. There was no need to put Him in the middle of this mess now, right?

God put Himself smack in the middle of my son's destiny. After giving Macey my final *no* on having a baby inconvenience my career, I fell into a deep sleep. I was feeling really good about not having to go forward with the struggles of raising a child. I could have lost my scholarship and starting position on the basketball team, and what seemed to be the worse part of this whole fix was losing my banging body where my six-pack was proudly showcased. You would think I would have had these thoughts prior to getting pregnant.

That night, I had a dream that the sun was shining and someone had provided me with the money I needed to pay for the procedure. I was on the way to the abortion clinic. As I approached the double glass doors at the entrance to the clinic, I heard a quiet voice say to me: "Don't touch that baby, he's ordained." I wanted what I wanted, and my mind was made up; my spirit, which could have intervened, was asleep right along with my body. Still dreaming, I proceeded. The voice and the command got louder and louder as I approached the entrance. Finally, the sky went dark and wind began to blow as the command became a demand. I was crippled in my process, brought to my knees, then overwhelmed by a fear of God that had lay dormant since I was a child in vacation Bible school. I was awakened along with my spirit that night. I sat up in that hotel bed with my eyes filled with tears. I saw a bright light in the ceiling of the pitch-black room, and I was totally conscious and exclaiming, "I won't, I won't." Macey was awakened by the cry. He asked what was wrong and who I was talking to. After all that we have been through, we still remember that night.

Spiritual Jeopardy

To become responsible parents without losing our scholarships, we got married without counsel or prayer or wisdom. God still honored us. We were blessed and highly favored in that situation just because God is faithful. The marriage in and of itself struggled, but the partnership we established is even stronger today than it was back then. Even though I had no idea what it meant to be a wife, I knew that marriage was supposed to be special and forever, like we had said in our vows, until death parted us. We were not supposed to be separated by infidelity and misunderstandings. We were supposed to make it through those challenges.

We ruled in our sports. Marriage should have been a piece of cake. It was not. It was closer to a recurring nightmare. I was devastated and empty when Macey and I separated for the first time. I really did not know what to do, so I did what most women do: I kept falling back into the Nightmare on Elm Street because that was most familiar to me. The relationship never got better because, just like in the battle with the bulge, the underlying issues were never dealt with. We just wanted to be together, like some people just want to lose weight, but we never counted the cost of a successful marriage and perhaps never had the resources to fully cover the expenses. I had many struggles as a child reared in a single parent home, challenges in sports competitions, even getting back into school after missing an entire year and earning my position back on the team. Surely I could win at a relationship initiated with so much love, hope, and possibilities.

Spiritual Divorce

Christ is Love. Without Him, my relationship and marriage fell apart, and I was left in a vulnerable state. I attended summer school and finished my degree on time, just as my marriage was ending. After graduation, I was exhausted. My top-notch body and razor-sharp mind were spent. I had nothing left. I was empty. I was running on the fumes of my mother's prayers and God's amazing grace. I would eat and sleep. The spirit of depression settled on me. I was spiritually empty. I had no sword of the spirit, which is the Word of God—the only offensive weapon we are allotted, according to Scripture. There I was with not even a butter knife (spiritually speaking), but a plastic disposable knife from what I had learned about Scripture in vacation Bible school. I was in trouble.

I became inactive because I had no desire to do anything after I finished my college basketball career. Remember, we practiced "in and out of season." Oh, but if I had known to put a fraction of that time and energy into strengthening my spirit as much as I did sharpening my body and skill set, this testimony would be obsolete. Thank God, for this testimony gave me a foundation full of compassion and understanding that I could not have obtained any other way.

Then, the rains came, the wind blew and the floods descended upon me and my household. We were divided, at odds, in constant disagreement. We did not attend church, study God's word, or pray together. So we did not stay together. If we, as a couple, not just me or him, but *we*, had had a firm foundation in Jesus Christ, we would have lasted the storms that hit our home. Our lives were spared, and our destinies are still coming to fruition, but the impact of the attack on our marriage left us both spiritually devastated.

We agree that our speedy healing and recovery was directly linked to our individual bloodline covenants set in order by our parents. We came from firm spiritual foundations that saved us, if not the marriage. Thank God for His enduring covenant even over the children of those who love Him and fearfully worship Him. Even if you or a family member is not in a personal relationship with God, a covenant family relationship filled with His promises can still offer covering and protection. My mother's relationship with the Lord Jesus Christ and her faith in Him protected me and trained me up in the ways of God to which I would eventually return. Hallelujah! Thank you, Jesus! That is so important and so powerful. God always keeps His covenants. God honored His covenant with my mother, Dorothy Vassell, just as He honored His covenant with Abraham, Isaac, and Jacob. (See Exodus 2:24-25.)

Spiritual Drought

Less than a year later, I was totally out of money, energy, and a marriage. I became ill in my body because I was spiritually dehydrated. My phone was off and there was no gas in my 1979 Toyota Celica that only started occasionally. There was someone that I could have called, but I had no way to call her. I was sick. I was really sick all the way around. I did not have any cold medicine or a way to call for someone to help get me some. It was me and my son, who was three years old at the time, and our two bedroom, one bath, shotgun style apartment. I felt like I would die and no one would know to come and get me and take care of Dontre. I felt like I was dying.

Now, I am glad that I was in that place because that place threatened my spirit and caused it to cry out to God and challenge His authority and power over my life. I remember saying to the Lord, "If you are real and you can help me, I need you right now to show up and deliver me." I got up, went into the kitchen to get a glass of water, and I must have passed out on the kitchen floor. I was so weak. Hallelujah! God is made strong in our weakness. I do not recall anything, not even passing out. I just remember regaining consciousness as Dontre sat beside me in silent reverence for what was happening to me.

I often wonder if he was praying for me, or if he saw something. He never said anything to me about it. He was only three years old. I don't recall being shaken or touched. He was just standing there when I came to.

I have never been the same since that day. It was as if God performed surgery on my spirit. I was no longer sick. I was healed. My heart felt new and my perception had changed. It was as if some sort of cloudiness was removed, and I could feel the richness of the atmosphere. My mind was not the same. I could finally fill my spirit. A few hours later, a professor who had attempted to contact me by phone from the university, one who was familiar with my work, used my school address and stopped by my tiny apartment to offer me an adjunct faculty job that would pay $4,000 that same month. I was astonished. My life has never been the same. Affliction will not rise up a second time (See Nahum 1:9).

Spiritual Plateau

Even after this experience, the weight continued to pile on. I gained pound after pound, and I did not even know I was fat until my clothes stopped fitting. I went to join a gym only to find that I had gained over thirty pounds in six months. I went from an athletic 160 pounds to 192 pounds. I am 5'10". All of that weight was in my hips and thighs, and I was as wide as all outside. My mouth dropped in disbelief as former classmates and teammates watched from a distance at the downward turn my life had taken. I went home and stood in front of my mirror, and I exclaimed to myself that I was not going to be two hundred anything, and I meant it with all that was in me.

Spiritual Restoration

Although I had been delivered from spiritual barrenness, I was still carrying lots of emotional baggage that translated into spiritual heaviness. I did not know the yoke-breaking and stronghold-tearing-down power of the blood of Jesus Christ, coupled with praise and worship, like I do now. I began to exercise and work out in the gym about three hours a day, but, this time, I also added a massive personal study of the Word of God every morning at the banks of the Edisto River in Orangeburg, South Carolina.

After four months, I had lost only four pounds, physically. I was hit hard and hurt by the results of a quarter of a pound per week. At that time, I am not sure what my body fat percentage or muscle weight was. I was putting in a lot of physical effort, but lacked some solid principals and fundamental knowledge. I just knew I could no longer fit in my clothes.

God was faithful to me because I was adding prayer and a daily intake of His Word in my life, and I could tell the difference in my perspective. While my eyes were fixated on the scale, God was establishing a just balance in my spirit. I was having a spiritual workout that would literally change my outlook on lots of things in my life. I discussed the weight loss issues I was having with some of the girls from the gym I had joined. They gave me a simple challenge to watch everything I ate, especially foods with a high fat content. Historically, I ate whatever I wanted to eat as an athlete with no respect for nutritional value or balance. I assumed this was the way things would work for me once again. It was not working at all. I was older, and my level of activity was greatly reduced. Even the top fitness experts do not hold an exercise regimen comparable to college athletes.

I took the challenge, disciplined my mouth, organized my meals every day and refused to eat high-calorie foods and sweets. I turned down invitations to lunch or dinner that fell outside of my eating schedule, and, within two months, I had lost the entire thirty pounds. My metabolism was high because of all of the exercise I had been doing over the four-month period. The problem was that I had been canceling out all of my caloric loss with excessive caloric intake. I had been breaking even. As soon as I made the adjustment in my diet, the weight came off, and I felt like I had my life back for the first time in years. Some form of fitness had been a mainstay the majority of my life, but not faith. This had cost me a high price, emotionally and interpersonally. Hallelujah to the Most High for enlightenment.

Since that time, much has changed: addresses, phone numbers, relationships, faces, towns, jobs, and careers. A lot has changed. But there are two things that have remained the same and have kept me healthy, strong, and growing in Christ amidst some very severe storms in my life: My faith and fitness.

Spiritual Submission

So, where are you spiritually? If you are overweight, can you pinpoint exactly what triggered the weight gain? Was it a pregnancy? Did you begin a new job? Was it due to an injury? Perhaps you have had weight challenges all of your life. Whatever your plight is, it does not have to remain that way. One major consistency that I have observed in dealing with clients who have found great success in overcoming obstacles associated with being fit and healthy is that they are spiritually grounded in a relationship with the Lord Jesus Christ. They have wholeheartedly subscribed to a walk of total forgiveness. And they trust wholeheartedly in the Word of God. They have turned from the fad diets of the world and embraced the temperance and self-control of the Holy Spirit.

You can too. You can master your mind and spirit by bringing them both under the submission of the Holy Spirit. Greater is He, the literal Spirit of God that lives in you, than any remedies the world could possibly substitute. You will learn through the spirit of truth how to live and socialize in this world without becoming dependent on its compromised value system and anti-Christ attitude. You can thrive and win with Christ. Yes, you can, even in this unfriendly world of temptation and immorality. Be not overcome with evil, but overcome evil with good, which is God. (See Romans 12:21).

Jesus Christ has overcome the world. You have unlimited authority through Christ Jesus. We are seated with Him in heavenly places. This spiritual authority must be exercised in your own life and in the home before you are mature enough to attempt facing societal battles. Spiritual preparation begins with a mastering of yourself and the space you occupy, abiding under the shadow of the Most High God.

Survivor's Map

Use the space below to describe, as I did above, that time, place, and season when you lost yourself and never recovered. Take your time. Think clearly and recall your state of mind at that time. If you need extra space, use extra paper. Be sure to put any extra sheets in this space in the book right behind the prayer that follows.

"In order to find myself, I shall recall where I lost myself." –JW

_____
_____
_____
_____
_____
_____
_____
_____
_____
_____
_____
_____
_____

_____
_____
_____
_____
_____
_____
_____
_____
_____
_____
_____
_____
_____
_____
_____
_____
_____
_____
_____
_____
_____
_____
_____
_____

Spiritual Speech: Prayer

Father God, in the matchless name of Jesus Christ, we thank you that you did not leave us lonely and comfortless when you ascended back into the heavens in the form of the resurrected Christ. You sent us a great comforter and leader in the Holy Spirit. Father, teach us to be still and know that you are God. Teach us throughout the day that it is not by the power of our diminishing wills and minds that falter when we are weak or pressed, and it is not by our physical might that is challenged on every end and ultimately wiped out with the tests of time, but it is by your omnipotent, omniscient, and omnipresent Holy Spirit that we are kept until that perfect day when Christ returns. Some trust in chariots and some trust in horses, but we will remember the name of the Lord, our God. They are fallen, but we are risen and stand upright.

Lord, let the King of Glory hear us when we call. Help us to make a firm commitment to you and to ourselves to never become spiritually dormant again. Help us to keep our spirit filled with good things so that our spiritual weight is of strength and not of heaviness. In times of weakness, confusion, and uncertainty, help us to run to the rock of Jesus Christ. At all times, Father, let us dwell in the secret place of the Most High and abide under the shadow of the Almighty. Let us say that you are our rock and our refuge and our fortress, our God.

Create in us a clean mind, a clean body, and renew a right spirit within us. We surrender our spirits to you, oh Lord. Shine through us and bless those around us. We lay aside every weight that besets us, and we embrace your way of ease and light burdens. We thank you that your blessings and way makes us prosperous in all aspects of our lives and adds no sorrow. Be glorified in our lives, oh God. Be magnified in all that we are and all that you plan for us to be. We worship you in spirit and in truth.

Father God, as I gather the broken pieces of my spirit, I bring them to you, the potter of my soul, to put them back together again. I have pointed out times and events that caused me to lose sight of who I am in you. Thank you, Father God, that nothing is ever lost in your eyes. You have been with me the entire time, and you know my beginning from my end. Lord, I submit this event of my past that shook my life to you.

Thank you, Lord. You are the God of second chances. Teach me to be faithful in this new opportunity to become fit and healthy. You know the plans that you have for me. Do with me as you please. I trust you with my whole heart. Hallelujah! Oh Glory! Hallelujah! Amen!

Surviving the Body Shaping Game: Master Building

"For we are labourers together with God: ye are God's husbandry, ye are God's building. According to the grace of God which is given unto me, as a wise masterbuilder, I have laid the foundation, and another buildeth thereon. But let every man take heed how he buildeth thereupon" (1 Corinthians 3:9-10).

A "Triangle" Building: Mind, Body, Soul

God is our Master Builder. He has already built our houses, temples, and bodies, and His craftsmanship is unparalleled by even the most complex computer, the smartest car, or the highest flying rocket. Please note that you, God's handiwork, are made in His very own image. You have been given power to rule, reign, create, and subdue. All of those gifts are man's when using the wisdom and knowledge of God. Your body is a fine-tuned machine, driven by the forces and intentions of the mind and fueled by the spirit. Realizing this is a vital step in developing a holistic balance in life. Most people start with the body and ignore the key component of the mind and the spirit. The reason that I address the body last in preparation is because, ultimately, it has the least amount of power or control. Yet, its role is not to be ignored or denied.

Earlier, I mentioned that the last bit of personal accountability and self-restraint most people experience or use is within the confines of the career that now places food on the table. For others, this last bit was issued in their parents' home. Think about this. When you were a child, your parents controlled you. They did not control your mind or your spirit, but they controlled the actions of your body. Oh, if they really knew what you thought of those chores and the unsolicited advice they so often shared, you would be in big trouble, even now. What about your meals? You had no money, no job, and no way to get to a food establishment to get what you "wanted" to eat. You ate what was before you and, as a matter of fact, most of you ate all of it, or else! There were rules about when you drank, and that bit of dessert after dinner, if any, might be taken away with an altercation at the table or the slightest misbehavior. You did not "like" it, but you dealt with it, and it was for your own good.

Baby Buildings

It is your job to be a faithful steward over that which God has entrusted you. You must watch over your marriage, your children, your career, and your mind, spirit, and body. Besides, no one could do all of this with grace and love like you. As a society, we are faithful and diligent in keeping our country pristine and filled with the latest advancements. The United States of America leads the world in executing the power to rule, reign, create, and subdue. However, somewhere between the compounded knowledge we have accumulated in our libraries and universities and the advancement of computer technology through fiber optics, we have lost perspective on our health. While leading the world in several impressive categories, we also lead the world in obesity, inactivity, diabetes, cancer, heart disease, and, it would be safe to assume, divorce, depression, heartache, and pain. These are only a few of the known categories based on the most recent data (www.cdc.gov).

In the last decade, there have been over two million pharmacies opened. Pharmacies are conveniently situated in supermarkets and department stores, and, nowadays, there is one on just about every street corner. We have gained more knowledge, but less perspective. Childhood obesity is thoughtfully mentioned as a charitable cause here and there, but this epidemic is a stronghold that will be very difficult to break for our youth once they reach adulthood.

Think of this: ten to twenty years ago, there was not much mention of childhood obesity on a national scale. However, today adults twenty and older who *were not obese children* struggle with weight loss and making good food choices. So what will be the future of the many obese children of today? These children are not just husky or holding a few pounds of baby fat. Inactivity and diets saturated with sugar and bad fats have caused their body composition to move from obese to morbidly obese. Without intervention, not only will children be more than likely to suffer from a poor quality of life in childhood, but a short lifespan can be expected. Not only must we start taking authority over our own bellies and bodies holistically, we must intervene for entire generations of men, women, and children who do not know better.

Building Violation: Four-Letter Words

So, what happened to all of that structure and discipline? You would think that you would have adopted some of that home training and actually used it as an adult. On the contrary, most of you could not wait to leave home so you could finally do whatever you "felt" like doing. What a tragedy, because the body needs structure and discipline. Without it, the body will run itself ragged, and that is not good. Without structure and focus, the body will do three "red zone" things: exactly what it "likes, wants, and feels."

When my clients use any of these three words, I remind them that these are elementary school words that have no place in personal training. "I don't *like* this exercise." "I *want* some cheesecake. Come on, just a small piece." "I don't *feel* like working out today. Can I reschedule?"

I have heard it all, and I continue to hear more excuses every day. Imagine a life driven by what a person likes, wants, or feels. Of course we go to work every day to pay the bills and take care of our families. Being undisciplined does not make us irresponsible or stupid. Most of the time, we make sure that our homes are reasonably clean and organized. We are not slobs. We would never forsake the fellowship with our church families. This would be blasphemous. So here we are with a firm grasp of mastering all of these external prerequisites. We are functioning and doing better than most, but even this is killing us, for our mouths and flesh are out of control.

Building Habits

One of my clients enlisted his wife and three daughters in my fitness program once school was out for the summer. He was determined that his girls would be healthy and strong. One of the girls showed the potential of being relatively overweight consistent with her genetic profile. This disturbed her father, as he refused to see his daughter share the fate of his sisters and mother. His family had a history of obesity associated with poor eating habits and inactivity. His sisters each had high blood pressure, obesity, and he had recently lost one of them to an asthmatic attack at their parents' home. I mentored the girls as we trained, shopped, and participated in various extracurricular activities. We had a great relationship. I found that they were on a very restricted diet. This was a very harsh diet, extremely unrealistic for children. The girls' dad had come up with this diet. I do not recommend diets for school-aged children. I suggest supplementing their diets with more fruits and vegetables.

The girls revealed the funniest thing to me. I was addressing a negative behavior that was revealed to me by the father. He told me that she was sneaking snacks and being rebellious. I asked the girls where they found the snacks, and they said they were the father's snacks. I was shocked. He had his own stash of cookies, chips, and candies that the girls would find and eat no matter how hard he tried to hide them. How could he do this to his daughters? I told him, "You cannot do that. You are the adult and you must lead by example." He excused himself, stating that he did not eat them often, just every now and then. If he had simply set an example of a healthy lifestyle as opposed to teaching them one way and living his life another way, his daughters would have accepted the lifestyle. Everyone would have been healthier and happier. He was a hypocrite in the eyes of his daughters.

Being a Better Building

The client "knew" what he wanted for his children, but he lacked the physical discipline to implement his own philosophy of healthy food choices into his daily routine. Your body is innately adaptive. This means that you can break or make any habit with a plan, theoretically, in twenty-one days or less. Your body is designed for self-preservation, healing, and self-maintenance. Whatever you want your body to do, all you have to do is expose it, train it, and reinforce it. It will follow whatever plan you wish, negative or positive.

Every person you meet is a byproduct of the habits that he or she has formed or broken. The word *habitual* is a serious word. Talking, eating, drinking, lying, procrastination, exercising, bragging, reading, drinking coffee, smoking, worship, charity, singing—all of these can be considered habits of human nature. This is an indication that the body can be trained to do whatever our mind and spirit tells it to. This is where mind over matter really becomes significant and the spirit must settle all arguments that arise between the body and the mind.

Once we establish the fundamental principles that the body must follow, we must not give in to its whimpers, complaints, or its desire to compromise. We must treat ourselves like children enforcing mandatory policy and procedures for eating and exercising, no matter what we want, like, or feel from day to day. As it was when we were children, this is for our own good.

The Building Buzz

Physical preparation begins with forcing your body to comply. Your conscience wants you to be successful and do the right thing, but your body wants to do what it feels like doing, or what it is familiar with doing. Here are some examples of actively bringing the body under submission:

1. Folding that basket of clothes that has been sitting there all week.

2. Eating that salad when you really want a fried chicken sandwich.

3. Emptying the dishwasher each night.

4. Not eating in your car.

5. Not eating unless you take time to cook or make your own meal. Big challenge!

6. Thanking God *every day* for ten or more blessings.

7. Recording events and hopes for the future daily.

8. Not eating meat for a week. Not eating sweets for a week.

9. Not watching television more frequently than two days each week.

10. Thinking before speaking in every conversation, and only commenting positively.

Your Own Building Code

This is a random list to give you an idea of how to begin commanding your flesh and preparing it for optimal living. Some of the items on the list above may not apply to your situation, but I am sure that you can easily create a list that applies to you. This is a small yet effective method of controlling your body instead of your body controlling you. Once you know better, do better. You'll do better when you develop a balance between your mind, body, and spirit, granting dominance to the latter. On rare occasions, the mind gives into the flesh and disaster is almost always the outcome. This is what we must overcome. This is why we are laying the groundwork for fitness with mind and spirit preparation. If your mind is clean, firm, and Christlike, and the Holy Spirit commands *your* spirit, then they will both diligently fight for what is in the best interest of the body.

Building Brainstorm

Let's brainstorm and think back to a time and place when you were at your best. If you have a picture that captured a period of your life when you were thinner, happier, and more focused, find it for this exercise.

Place the picture on your mirror, in your Bible, in this devotional or somewhere so that you can see where you once were and want to be. Also, in addition to your glamour shot from the past, gather a recent picture, one taken within the past thirty days. If you don't have a picture, don't be ashamed to take one now. Even if it is just your belly that you are working on, once you are blessed, God deserves His glory through your testimony. Many are moved by the testimony of one. Do not be ashamed! God is up to the task. The bigger the job, the bigger the blessing, and the more sincerely you may praise Him. God is about to gain glory for himself by doing a new thing in your life, and you will help others overcome by the word and pictures of your testimony.

Get ready! We are asking God to do a new thing in your life, as only He can. Keep that photo close by, for you will soon see that your latter days will be greater than your former days. The best is yet to come.

Blessing the Building: Prayer

Father God, I know that my body is the temple of the Holy Spirit. Lord, send your Holy Spirit to move, breath, and live in my physical body. I know that my spirit is willing, but my flesh is weak. I acknowledge that I am weak-willed and often tempted to do and say things that are contrary to your will for my life. Thank you for your mercy and grace and for allowing me the option to overcome by the blood of the Lamb.

I know that faith without works is a dead faith. Help me to demonstrate my faith in the discipline and work manifested through my earthly body. My body is the tool you have equipped me with to bring forth offspring created

in your image. My body is what I use to help those in need, serve your people, and bring you the sacrifice of worship. Help me to be a faithful steward over my physical body and overall health, taking full advantage of each and every day here on Earth with which I am blessed.

I know that I am made from dust, and to the dust I will return. Until then, Father, make me complete, a perfected creature to bring glory to your name and honor to your throne. I want to look like our heavenly Father in word, action, and deed. You are mighty, Father God. With us, this looks impossible, but with you, God, all things are possible. Show us the possibilities of a body ruled by your Holy Spirit and enhanced by the substance of your Holy Word. Hallelujah! Oh Glory! Hallelujah! Amen!

Confessional Conclusion

Each day that I turn on the television or log in on my computer, I see another advertisement to "help" Americans lose weight. There are so many weight loss supplements and products on the market that the average consumer may have to take a mini-course to fully understand them all. There is more exercise equipment on the market than there has ever been before. There is an equal amount of equipment stored in the houses of those who purchase it with the hopes of losing weight. Excess weight is not gained overnight, thus there is no quick fix. As a matter of fact, quick weight loss is not only dangerous, but it is almost always temporary.

Your health is your wealth and the vehicle to your destiny. Not only have I seen many bodies transformed through the weight loss and fitness process, but I have seen lives transformed and dreams fulfilled. Your body will be with you for the rest of your life. Your body should be "kept" in optimal condition. I am not sure if you are overweight in your body or in your spirit, but a strong command of the "triangle" (body, mind, spirit) will blaze a path in your life like you have never seen. The growth and strengthening process outlined in this book may be used to overcome just about any challenge or obstacle that you may face.

Weight loss has been turned into a huge game of counting calories, exercising, joining the biggest gym and taking the right weight loss products. There is a game of eating fewer carbohydrates and more proteins. There is a game of eating six times a day, and another that dismisses food all together. There is the bulimic game. There is the game of gastric bypass surgery.

Please do not play games with your life. What profits a man to lose twenty pounds and gain cancer or liver damage? What profits a woman to loss fifty pounds at the expense of esophagus erosion and stomach damage? Why play games with your life? You do not have to play these games. While we believe that we have the victory over death, sickness, disease, and every attack of the enemy, we must realize that we have authority over the weight-related issues in our lives. God has given us authority over our entire beings. We have authority over our minds. We have authority over our spirits. We have authority over our cravings. We have authority over our bodies. We only have to train ourselves and practice actively walking in that authority.

I know what it is like to be spiritually grounded. I know what it is like to have a sound, stable mind. I know what it is like to execute discipline in control of the body. However, it is only through the combined force of the three that total victory is achieved, no matter what game is played. You are on your way to never having to struggle with weight loss, or any loss, again.

As I once said on *The Early Show*: "Sometimes, when you win, you really lose, and, when you lose, you really win." In all that you have experienced and all that you think it cost you, you are now prepared for the next level. Be brave and have faith. Live and take authority. Life can be a jungle of futility, but with the right training and preparation you can survive the game.

PART 2

"Peaces"
of the
PINEAPPLE

28 Day
Devotional Workout

Introduction

God is omnipotent, omniscient, and omnipresent. This means that God has unlimited authority and influence. He is all-powerful and almighty at the same time. Because God is also omniscient, He has infinite awareness, understanding, and insight. He knows all things and is infinitely wise. How is this? Omniscient means to be *exhaustively* learned. There is no more knowledge for God to acquire. He is capable of appearing everywhere at once. Hallelujah! What a mighty God we serve. There is great security and assurance in trusting God.

David exclaims, "Bless the Lord, O my soul, and all that is within me, bless his holy name. Bless the Lord, O my soul, and forget none of his benefits" (Psalm 103:2, NASB). David is telling us that there are benefits to serving, praising, worshiping, and obeying an omnipotent, omniscient, and omnipresent God, and we need to remember this.

Trust

We can trust in the Lord our God because He is all-knowing, wise, and within all places at all times. He is the God who knows your beginning and your end. He knows your enemies and your friends. He knows what you can handle and what you cannot handle. God's plan for your life cannot fail. This does not make it any easier to step out in faith and move in the direction of the things for which God has called you.

Abraham, in Genesis Chapter 12, displays an unwavering faith by leaving family and familiarity to enter a place God would show him. In return, God promised Abraham that he would be blessed, he would become a blessing, and he would become a great nation.

"Now the Lord had said unto Abram, Get thee out of thy country, and from thy kindred, and from thy father's house, unto a land that I will shew thee: And I will make of thee a great nation, and I will bless thee, and make thy name great; and thou shalt be a blessing" (Genesis 12: 1-2).

God honors Abraham's obedience and indeed blesses him to become a blessing as indicated in the earned name change of Abraham. Two parts of the threefold promise had been fulfilled. There was still more, and Abraham and Sarah, even in their old age, were made to receive the later part of the promise. Isaac, who would become a great nation, was born to Abraham and Sarah, who had basically given up on ever having a child. God did exactly what He said He would do. And, however imperfect he was, Abraham moved when God said *move*. As a result, his family was blessed. Abraham is further tested when the child of promise is born to his wife Sarah in her old age.

Ten chapters later, in Genesis Chapter 22:2, Abraham's obedience and faith are tested once again. God requests that Isaac, Abraham's son, his only son, whom he loves, be offered up to him as a burnt sacrifice. Was God's promise that Abraham would father a great nation now being retracted? YES—Isaac's death would be the death of Abraham's only seed. Yes. Again, without consultation, question, delay another day, calling a church prayer meeting or a twenty-one-day fast, Abraham simply obeys God.

"And it came to pass after these things, that God did tempt Abraham, and said unto him, Abraham: and he said, Behold, here I am. And he said, Take now thy son, thine only son Isaac, whom thou lovest, and get thee into the land of Moriah; and offer him there for a burnt offering upon one of the mountains which I will tell thee of" (Genesis 22:1-2).

Faith and Obedience

Is faith and obedience as simple as Abraham made it seem? Abraham was seventy-five years old when God told him to "get out." He had to walk away from all of his friends and relatives. He had to leave all of his personal and professional contacts. He had to leave his possessions and personal property. Abraham simply obeyed God, and this was the costly fuel of his destiny. There are very few people who have the blind faith and sacrificial obedience of Abraham.

Has God ever given you a specific command that lingered on your heart for many days and you simply ignored His pull at your heartstrings? A great destiny requires great sacrifice. God is sensitive to our overstretched and stressed plights, so He often makes simple requests that we can handle: love, fast, pray, exercise, give, forgive, apologize, read, study, speak, keep silent, testify, stay, go, let go, rest.

Do these sound familiar? Even with our great example of Abraham and the faithfulness God has shown us deliberately over the years, we still find it difficult to simply obey God. The inability to tap into an awaited destiny through the revelation of an all-knowing, wise God who knows the beginning to the end may be a result of fear, uncertainty, doubt, or past failures.

Moving Forward

Fear, failure, doubt, and uncertainty are huge inhibitors when it comes to moving forward and achieving one's destiny. As I boldly entered the final stages of the audition process to become one of sixteen contestants on the hit reality TV show "Survivor," I was tested. You could say that I had an Abraham experience, and I almost forfeited my promise. Fortunately, the call on my life was so vital that God sent me great counsel as I matured in life and in my walk with Him.

My mother, Evangelist Dorothy Vassell, was my greatest confidant and source of reference and wisdom. She was my friend and my teacher. My mother had watched and prayed over many transitions in my life. She had not only witnessed the highs and lows of my thirty years, but she also prayed and fasted for me on many occasions. The stringent application process for "Survivor" was nothing compared to the challenges I faced in college as a student athlete, parent, and wife. It was nothing compared to the painstaking marriage that led to a divorce only a few years earlier. I was as bold as a lion, for I had seen the power of faith, prayer, fasting, and agreement. Nothing could stop me. No matter how I was challenged or what came my way, I had already survived great feats. This boldness was embedded in a tested, tried, and true faith in God and constant support and insight from one of the greatest modern-day prophets I knew.

My mother was so excited and full of prophecy about my participation in the game. I was very confident because I had been down this road before. If God brought me to it, certainly He was able to bring me through it. As usual, my mother had committed herself to fasting and praying for me throughout this process. I had been here before and I knew that the outcome would be favorable again. In the middle of the month, as I sat at my desk in the guidance suite at my school, I received a call from the producers of the show telling me that I was a finalist for the show. I immediately called to share the news with my mother who began to glorify God for showing her daughter so much favor.

Final Phase

I would have to leave for the final audition phase in only a few weeks and preparations had to be secretly made in keeping with the rules of the show. My mother, friend, and confidant would oversee my affairs while I departed from my well-balanced life filled with praise and worship, church and Bible study, exercise and recreation, friends and family. My life, at that time, had recently been transformed from major drama and confusion to peace and restitution, and we both marveled at all that was happening. In that same month, I got another phone call as I was leaving a late-night aerobics class. This phone call would not only change my life but my entire destiny. It was my brother-in-law telling me that my mother had passed away only hours earlier.

In disbelief, I dropped the call and called each of my mother's phones, and she did not answer. She had always answered. This was the most devastating moment of my life. Up till then my confidence and blessed assurance had laid in the solace that while the body was attainable, my spirit and soul belonged to God. On that night, my mother's death had an effect on my entire being. I was filled with grief and despair as I experienced my first and only spiritual blow. I was hit with a right-left combination of grief, fear, and despair. My fingertips began to numb and my body began to tremble. I broke out in hives and could not eat. As a seasoned student of the Bible, I knew firsthand that God gave life and took it away. I knew that the blood of His saints was precious in His eyes, and to be absent with the body was to be one with God. But what about all of those hopes, expectations, and unfulfilled promises my mother expressed?

Faith for the Challenge

During one of our usual daily discussions only the day before, I had shared with my mother how I stood my ground when the CBS staff member called to challenge my faith and my ability to survive the harsh environments of the show locations. I assured the staff that earth was the Lord's and all that was in it, and therefore I would be taken care of. I spoke confidently and brashly to the staff about my faith and trusted in the Lord. I remember that the final question on that day from the caller was, "And you trust God like that?"

I recall this part of our last conversation the day before she passed. "Mama," I said, "I told them, I am not afraid. I trust God. They just don't know how faithful our God is, do they? I wonder sometimes if God really knows how much I trust Him."

My mother replied, gently, "Well, Nahum 1:7 states that God is a good God, and a stronghold in the day of trouble, and He knows those who trust in Him. He knows that you trust in Him, JoAnna." This was a conversation that I will never forget.

Physically strong, but spiritually crushed, I attended the funeral with my six siblings. This was the saddest group of individuals I had ever seen. Our mother was our rock and a direct reference point of our faith in God. The day after my mother's funeral, in the early morning hours, fear tapped me on the shoulder and confronted me with very realistic questions. I could not call my mother, my prayer partner, my best friend, my pastor. We had buried her the day before. I could only call on the Lord Jesus Christ.

I sat on the side of the bed. What would I do? Who would keep my son and maintain my balanced life? I thought, "Oh my God, my faith is on the line and everyone is watching to see what I am really made of." I was truly afraid for the first time in my life. I was stuck between a rock of fear and a hard place of faith and destiny. I opened the nightstand drawer and I pulled out the Gideon Bible. Prayer was not enough. I needed a word from the Lord himself. Nothing less would do. I needed to know that it was Him speaking not only to me, but to my tragic situation. I came to Isaiah 41:10. This scripture changed my life and has sustained me in making what I call "Abrahamic" decisions of destiny. This is my anthem:

"Fear thou not; for I am with thee: be not dismayed; for I am thy God: I will strengthen thee; yea, I will help thee; yea, I will uphold thee with the right hand of my righteousness" (Isaiah 41:10).

This is my interpretation of what I read in the hotel room early that morning:

"Do not be afraid. Your mother is with me. She was my daughter long before she became your mother. She is resting now. Do not be afraid. I am here with you and I will be with you in whatever you do. I am YOUR God. I belong to you and you belong to me. I know that you are weak, but I will strengthen you. Do not be afraid to leave your son with me, your only son, whom you love. I spared him from your own hand when you were a confused college athlete. I have taken care of both of you, haven't I?

"Do not be afraid. I will make you stronger through this experience than you have ever been. I will cause your faith to be increased and your trust to lie ONLY in me. Go! Yes, I am with you. Go! Yes, I will help you with interviews, questions, and whatever you face. Go! I gave you the education and I provided you the job. I know how to take care of my own. Only trust me. You will lack nothing. Go! Yes, I will uphold you with my very own right hand. Go and I will reveal this plan to you, day by day. Trust me and go.

A Million Dollar Experience

I fell into a deep sleep and awoke to a frozen state of psychological, emotional, and spiritual dependence on God. My life and faith have never been the same. At the end of the final audition, I was chosen as one of the sweet sixteen for the next season of the show. Like Abraham, I was commissioned to go, and I did not know at the time that I boarded the airplane that I would lift my eyes in a land that I knew not.

The jungle of the Amazon rainforest was only a place that I had read about in geography class and seen in movies. To think, even as late as a day earlier, that I would live on the floor of the Amazon jungle literally amazed me. I was in a place of richness and wealth. I was in a place that reigns as the world's largest oxygen supply. This was an immaculate and beautiful place full of much healing, life, and, of course, dangerous predators. Black rivers, white sands, pink dolphins, anaconda, piranha, sting ray, electric eels, all add to the color and zeal of the jungle. While it sounds good on paper, the jungle is a creepy and dark place when you have been accustomed to electricity, running water, hot showers, a refrigerator, and a bed. This was survival of the fittest. One million dollars was the prize offered by the show. Thus, my greatest predators were the very people of my tribe that I slept with, ate with, and helped to survive. The glitz and glamour and the excitement of the show was flattering, as was the potential million dollar prize, but I had suffered great loss and expected restitution in a major way from God.

After my first few days in the steamy hot jungle situated only a stone's throw from the equator, I began to crave pineapples. This was not uncommon, as each one of us expressed a deep craving for some sort of food after involuntarily fasting on a diet of manioc and river water. It was so hot. I have never been so hot in my life. Unlike my tribe mates who eventually gave up on getting their craving filled before leaving the game, I continued to make my request known: "I sure would like some pineapple." My teammates assured me that the chance of me finding some pineapple out in the middle of the massive jungle was slim to none. They assured me that even if there were some pineapples in the jungle, the chance of them outlasting the consuming wildlife and making it to my lips would take place only in the form of a miracle.

Pineapples in the Jungle

This craving would not go away. I sang and worshipped God while in that jungle. Although everyone thought I was crazy and having psychotic reactions to the heat and starvation, I had firmly decided that my worship would protect and provide for me. My diligent partner and I rose early in the morning to hit the sticks in search of food and gaining a fundamental command of the jungle. We had to learn to respect even the daylight. The work hours and harvest hours lasted from sunup to sundown. The jungle is not a place to prowl around after dark. We had been out and about only a few hours on the day when, behold, we came across a hidden patch of jungle grass with two palm-sized pineapples. I screamed for so many reasons.

"Trust in the Lord, and do good; so shalt thou dwell in the land, and verily thou shalt be fed. Delight thyself also in the Lord; and he shall give thee the desires of thine heart. Commit

thy way unto the Lord; trust also in him; and he shall bring it to pass" (Psalm 37:3-5).

It was not berries or bananas that we found. We did not come across Brazil nuts or cornstalks. We found pineapples, the very food I had insistently craved amidst much skepticism. The very fruit that I said that I wanted was there, not just in the jungle, but in my hands! This was a Hallelujah moment! My partner and I jumped around and sang, and we were overwhelmed with the jewel of a fruit. We headed back to camp and slowly revealed our find. A hush went over our tribe as our tribe mates peered at the pineapples in disbelief and desire. Speechless, they could only wait to taste their small portion of a slice. This was the first and most profound of many miracles I experienced while I lived in the jungle. I emerged from the heat of the jungle on the twelfth day a renewed woman with an enhanced faith and opened eyes. The way that I experienced God and the changes He made in me could not be purchased with a billion dollars. The only acceptable exchange was faith and obedience.

We are all given a measure of faith coupled with a measure of disbelief. While my experience in the Amazon rainforest was a spiritual quest, it is not necessary to go through major extremes to simply obey God. So, what is preventing you from moving forth and getting out? Is it fear of the unknown that is holding you back? Are you concerned with what will happen to your children? What about that disease to please those around you and defending yourself from what they have to say about "God's" outrageous plan for your life?

I don't know what is holding you back, but I am familiar with "who" can bring you forth and provide you with many rams in the bushes of life. He did it for Abraham. He did it for me. For every vision, God gives a provision. God is omnipotent, omniscient, and omnipresent. You can trust God. He is faithful. He is an awesome God. He is Jehovah Jireh, the God who provides for you each and every day. There is nothing too hard for Him. Nothing is too complex or vast for Him. He is not only the master of your world, but He masters the universe. You can trust Him. We overcome by the blood of the Lamb and by the word of our testimony. God sent me all the way to the Amazon jungle with you in mind. He set in motion a provision of pineapples before I even know I would apply for the show. It takes up to eighteen months for a pineapple to mature for harvest.

"Peaces" of the Pineapple is our theme for this sweet, juicy, tasty, refreshing daily devotional that reminds us of God's constant provisions of love, peace, protection, direction, and everything else we need. No matter where you are or what God is calling you to do, great or small, He will provide you with everything you need for the journey. God constantly provides—even pineapples in the jungle.

Discipline in a "Foreign Land"

There are so many characters mentioned in the Bible that moved when God said to move. These biblical figures walked out their destiny driven by the voice of God, reinforced by relationships with God. There is, however, a group of guys whose courage and faith surpassed logic and understanding. I am referring to Hananiah, Mishael, and Azariah, who are also known as Shadrach, Meshach, and Abednego. These fellows displayed a remarkable faith and execution of discipline while in a foreign land.

Obviously, these young men had been taught the ways of the Lord. They opposed the king of the land at that time,

Nebuchadnezzar, who was known for cutting men into pieces and turning their homes into rubble. Although they opposed the king, it was not out of disrespect or arrogance. These were topnotch boys. They were the cream of the crop of the house of Judah. According to the book of Daniel, they were without blemish, well-favored, skilled in all wisdom and cunning in knowledge. In addition to the aforementioned traits, these children were obviously taught about the Lord and abhorred idol worship. With all respect and honor to the throne of the king, they were not "careful" in declining the king's offer to avoid the punishment of the fiery furnace by "simply" falling down and worshiping the golden image he had made. This is amazing:

*"Shadrach, Meshach, and Abednego answered and said to the king, O Nebuchadnezzar, we are not careful to answer thee in this matter. If it be so, our God whom we serve is able to deliver us from the burning fiery furnace, and he will deliver us out of thine hand, O king. **But if not, be it known unto thee**, O king, that we will **not** serve thy gods, nor worship the golden image which thou has set up"* (Daniel 3:16-18, emphasis mine).

How much courage and faith does it take to make a statement like that and to follow through with it when the heat of the furnace is on your face? What made them do it? They admitted that they knew God was able, but He had not disclosed to them that He would in fact save them from the fiery furnace. They were only sure of two things at this heated point of no return. They knew that God would deliver them from the king's hand, even at the cost of death, and they knew that they would not worship the king's gods or the golden image. They were immediately thrown into the fiery furnace, but the writer of Daniel tells us that not even the smell of fire was on them when they came out on the other side.

The Lord on My Side

I was confronted with a similar ultimatum while playing the game of Survivor in the Amazon jungle. I refused to acknowledge the presence of the "coveted" immunity idol that conveniently rested with only the winner of the day. I would not sit and sing around the fire with it. I would not lift it high in the air after leading my team to five out of six challenges. I knew better. Although my conviction was personal and not expected of my tribe mates, they could not understand my disdain for their "sweet" reward. I never chastised them for their homage of the lifeless image, but they questioned my position intensely. I was not moved by their arguments on behalf of the immunity idol. This line of questioning diminished after our first night with the idol because some really weird things began to happen in our makeshift—but otherwise harmonious—home.

One guy, a devout atheist, declared after one victory: "The Lord is on their side." Like the other men, he had never spoken to me, but they could feel and see the weaponry and warfare in my constant worship and giving glory to God in each challenge. I had no idea that they felt like "The Lord" was on our side until I saw the episodes. My stand about the idol became a national issue. Talk show hosts, listeners, and even "born-again believers" challenged my position of not touching the idol. Some people asked me, "How do you know that God will not be pleased if you touch the idol?" I declared without hesitation, "I am not absolutely sure if God will be pleased with me touching it or not, but just in case it displeases him, I am not going to touch it."

I felt something deep inside of me being grieved at the mere presence of that idol. That was the Holy Spirit leading me in the truth. I also felt that there was a spiritual significance to entering into covenant with it by touch and glorifying it at every victory. I felt like Eve in the garden, being told by the serpent,

"You will not surely die." I also recalled Uzzah's perilous fate as he reached to catch the Ark of God from falling. Although the Philistines had handled the Ark of God, it was forbidden for the children of Israel to touch it (2 Samuel 6:6).

God's Peace

So, what makes believers so bold in their faith to move when God says to move, to sacrifice long-awaited promises, to oppose violent and aggressive kings, to jeopardize a shot at a million dollar prize, or to shun the favor of Hollywood? It is God's peace. It is a peace that surpasses all understanding. It is a peace that the world does not give, because it cannot, and thus it cannot take the peace away. It is the peace of God. Seven is the number of both completion and perfection. The goal of this devotional is to help you find perfect peace with the completion of each week.

With this peace, you will be able to move forward in the things that God has ordained for your life. You will be able to give God your very best and move in complete obedience. When you face the Nebuchadnezzar of your life, you will have the peace and confidence to obey God and stick to His plan. When the heat is turned up "seven times" hotter in your life, and the famine of the jungle challenges your faith, you will walk with God and recognize that His righteous right hand will uphold you as He provides you sweet, succulent pineapples in the jungle.

"Peaces" of the Pineapple

Praise is comely and moves God.	**Spirit** of God is our Comforter.
Obedience is better than sacrifice.	**Sacrifice** produces destiny and deliverance.

Our 28-day devotional, "Peaces" of the Pineapple, is divided into four parts, each one week long. Each week covers a major fruit of maturity and lays a firm and well-balanced foundation for moving forward in the things of God. The major fruits of Christian life are Praise, Spirit, Obedience, and Sacrifice. At the end of these four weeks of perfection, you should find the strength to allow God to do His complete will in your life and to perfect His work in you.

"Though I walk in the midst of trouble, thou wilt revive me: thou shalt stretch forth thine hand against the wrath of mine

enemies, and thy right hand shall save me. The Lord will perfect
that which concerneth me: thy mercy, O Lord, endureth for ever:
forsake not the works of thine own hands" (Psalm 138:7-8).

Daily Disciplines

There are five daily disciplines to be practiced throughout
this devotional. They are the following: Promises of God,
Practice of the Word of God, Prayer, Power of Psalms, and a
Physical Activity.

The **Promises of God** are receipts that are good on the
return of God's Word. God backs His Word with a 100 percent
guarantee. It is important to keep all of your receipts with you
at all times. You never know when you will have to return to
God and remind Him of a promise He has made to you in His
Word. No matter how many times you have been let down,
disappointed, and lied to, God is not a man. He cannot lie. If
He promised or said something, that settles it, and it will be
so. Putting the **Word of God** into practice is vital. The Word
of God is the manufacturer's manual that we came with, and
we must follow the instructional guide in order to obtain our
purpose and live life to the fullest.

Prayer is how we communicate with God. Communication
with God is even more important than constant communication
with your spouse or family. God is the master of the universe.
Remember: He is omnipotent, omniscient, and omnipresent.
You will gain insight, wisdom, revelation, confirmation,
information, and guidance, just to name a few of the benefits
of communing daily with the all-knowing, wise, perfect God.
Do you want to know more about what is going on with your
children? Do you need to know more about who you are to
marry or if you are ready for marriage? Do you want to know

more about yourself? God has all of these answers and more. The good news is that He wants to share the answers with you.

"Call unto me, and I will answer thee, and shew thee great and mighty things, which thou knowest not" (Jeremiah 33:3).

The **Power of the Psalms** is a discipline that brings comfort, endurance, peace, and the abundance that God allocates for us. How do we prepare our residence for God? God inhabits the praises of His people. He lives in praise, worship, and adoration. Worship literally moves the heart of God.

David, as both a shepherd boy and King, sang praises and worshiped God. David has been adequately described as a man after God's own heart (Acts 13:22 and 1 Samuel 13:14). Thus, it does not come as a surprise that King David is a major contributor to the largest book of the Bible and this book happens to be filled with the magnificence and glory of the Most High God (El-Elyon). Even if we fast-forward to the end times and take a snapshot of God's throne, we see that God has surrounded himself with worship. *"They rest not day and night, saying, Holy, Holy, Holy, Lord God Almighty"* to God on His throne (Revelation 4:8-11). This level of adoration, while not making David perfect, did give him great favor, protection and influence with God. After David's death, God still honors His promises to David through his rebellious children.

Meditation on a Psalm a day is like taking a daily defense vitamin for your spirit.

"Speaking to yourselves in psalms and hymns and spiritual songs, singing and making melody in your heart to the Lord; Giving thanks always for all things unto God and the Father in the name of our Lord Jesus Christ" (Ephesians 5:19-20).

Exercise of the body is also important. **"Peaces" of the Pineapple** includes a daily **Physical Activity** that can be completed in as little as twenty minutes. The body is a vital tool in accomplishing destiny, serving others, and worshiping God. Physical activity also helps you to keep up with the pressures of life. Your body is the temple of the Holy Spirit, and it is the only vessel you have to engage in worshiping God. You will prosper and be in good health even as your soul prospers. Physical activity suppresses the appetite and reduces stress. It brings about an overall mood of euphoria and calmness.

The five daily disciplines will replenish and reassure the weak and weary soul, grant wisdom and resolution to life's issues, allow for ongoing communication with the master of the universe, demonstrate the most powerful and comforting Psalms, and will culminate with a strengthening and conditioning of the body through the daily discipline of physical activity. I hope that you are excited and ready for a change. This is your time. This is your season. This is all to the glory of God and meeting the destiny that He has in store for you.

Physical Activities

Before beginning any portion of the exercises outlined in this devotional, it is imperative that you have clearance from your medical doctor. If you suffer from extreme health problems, you are advised to share this outline with your doctor to ensure your ability to participate in these activities.

As you begin this 28-day devotional fitness program, there are a few items that I recommend you have. It is also necessary to designate a special area just for your daily devotional. Early morning, while the house is still quiet and others are asleep, you can set the atmosphere and the format of the day for yourself or for your entire family. The virtuous woman looks into the well-being of her household long before they even awake.

"She riseth also while it is yet night, and giveth meat to her household, and a portion to her maidens" (Proverbs 31:15).

By keeping your items together you will be able to access what you need from day to day without spending time in transition or looking for a piece of equipment. Here are the items you will need:

1. Cool water for each workout.
2. A hand towel.
3. A comfortable pair of walking/running shoes.
4. Two 10 lbs. hand weights. (Canned goods or water bottles will do initially.)
5. A workout mat. (A large towel will work, but watch your back.)
6. A jump rope.
7. A fitness ball. (55 cm or larger; it looks like an oversized beach ball)
8. A step, or clear access to stairs.
9. A chair.
10. Access to your favorite praise and worship music.

Always warm and stretch your muscles before doing any physically demanding activities. This includes some regular household chores. Here are sample warm-up and stretch activities:

1. **Warm-up**: March in place vigorously to your favorite up-tempo inspirational music, repeating the Promise and/or the Psalm discipline for the day, preferably aloud, for 4 minutes. Spend one minute meditating on each discipline. Three sets of 10 light jumping jacks is an adequate warm-up.

2. **Stretch**:
Shrug your shoulders backward and forward, tilting your head from side to side as you slowly turn your torso to your right and then to your left.

Standing with your legs apart and knees slightly bent, reach down to the right, then left, stretching for 15 seconds on each side.

Standing straight up, gently grasp your ankle or foot behind you to stretch your quadriceps for 15 seconds on each side.

Bending your elbow up with your hand behind your back, stretch your arms for 15 seconds on each side.

Understanding the Grid

In the first left column of the grid (pages 68-69), you will find an outline for the types of exercises you will use for the next 28 days—or prayerfully even longer. There are five numbered core areas of workout with five individual exercises for each core. For example, to follow the arm regiment for deltoids, I would look at core 3.4. The second column has the wording "Pre-max." The Pre-program Maximum record will allow us to determine how much conditioning you have gained over the next four weeks. Working with a friend or relative, you will record the number of core exercises you can do without stopping. For example, how long can you run (1.3) or jump a rope (1.4) without stopping? Using a stopwatch or timer for accuracy, you will record this time under "pre-max" next to (1.3) running and (1.4) jump rope. I will break down the differences between running, jogging, and walking in the definitions section.

Another way you will record your Pre-program Max will be by tracking repetition. For example, record the total number of crunches (4.2) you can do on your mat without stopping. The next four columns are to record your weekly progress. After the four weeks are completed, find the Total column. Use this column to record the total combined number of maximums from each week. There is also a Post-program Maximum column. The Post-Program Maximum should be recorded immediately after the completion of week four. No more than three days should elapse before you record your final program maximum. Compare your Pre-max and Post-max numbers. There should be a significant difference. This difference is called *fitness*. Each week, you should grow stronger and faster.

Fitness and Weight Loss

You should see your repetitions, duration, and overall endurance increase. Fitness should be our objective long before we seek any cosmetic benefits. A slender, well-toned body is a byproduct of fitness. Get fit and stay fit first, and then you will see the results you desire.

There is a distinct difference between weight loss and fitness. Not all weight loss is good. Millions of people experience weight loss due to involuntary starvation, while others experience weight loss due to mental, emotional, and physical illness. Thus, you should not become obsessed with the scale and the simplistic idea of losing weight to look better.

Your emphasis should be on trimming fat and becoming fit, because an obsession with weight loss could cloud the importance of vital muscle gain. Although muscle weighs more than fat, it burns more calories than fat. It also provides support for a stronger frame. When your frame is lined with lean muscle, you can endure longer work days with more zeal and energy

POWER

EXERCISE	Pre-Max	WEEK 1							WEEK 2						
		S	M	T	W	T	F	S	S	M	T	W	T	F	S
Core 1: CARDIO															
1. Walking															
2. Jogging															
3. Running															
4. Jump Rope															
5. Cardio Dance															
Core 2: LEG WORK															
1. Lunges															
2. Squats															
3. Glut Squeeze															
4. Leg Lifts															
5. Basic Step															
Core 3: ARM WORK															
1. Bi-cepts															
2. Tri-cepts															
3. Shoulders															
4. Deltoid lifts															
5. Chess Press															
Core 4: AB-WORK															
1. Basic Sit-ups															
2. Crunches															
3. Curl Crunch															
4. Hip Lifts															
5. Lying Peddle															
Core 5: BALL WORK															
1. Basic Crunch															
2. Full Fallback															
3. Pelvic Tilts															
4. Back Toner															
5. Oblique Toner															

GRID

EXERCISE	WEEK 3							WEEK 4							Total	Post-Max
	S	M	T	W	T	F	S	S	M	T	W	T	F	S		
Core 1: CARDIO																
1. Walking																
2. Jogging																
3. Running																
4. Jump Rope																
5. Cardio Dance																
Core 2: LEG WORK																
1. Lunges																
2. Squats																
3. Glut Squeeze																
4. Leg Lifts																
5. Basic Step																
Core 3: ARM WORK																
1. Bi-cepts																
2. Tri-cepts																
3. Shoulders																
4. Deltoid lifts																
5. Chess Press																
Core 4: AB-WORK																
1. Basic Sit-ups																
2. Crunches																
3. Curl Crunch																
4. Hip Lifts																
5. Lying Peddle																
Core 5: BALL WORK																
1. Basic Crunch																
2. Full Fallback																
3. Pelvic Tilts																
4. Back Toner																
5. Oblique Toner																

without caffeine and other drugs. Muscle also helps you sustain greater levels of impact from accidents.

Fitness Training DVD

Now that you've read this far, it's time to watch the DVD to learn our exercises. Please refer to p. 175, at the back of the book for **Descriptions and Instructions for Core Exercises.**

Week 1

Fruit of Praise

There are many ways to express adoration and appreciation. God, however, has outlined in His Word that those who worship Him must worship Him in spirit and in truth. Spirit and truth worship begins on an individual level with sincere thanksgiving for what God has done and for who He is.

Sincere congregational worship is a byproduct of intimate individual worship. There is a huge harvest of deliverance and freedom found in the fruit of worship. True worship ushers in the Holy Spirit of The Most High God. Once God shows up, hope springs forth and defeat and despair are subsequently eliminated.

In the next seven days, we will usher in the presence of the Holy Spirit through worship. These days of learning to worship include worshiping God even when it seems like all of the odds are stacked against you. There is nothing that activates the hand and heart of God like pure praise and worship. True worship is refreshing and spiritually invigorating. Once we learn the true power of constant praise and worship, we will literally see strongholds torn down, yokes broken, and the lives of those with whom we closely affiliate change.

"I will bless the Lord at all times: his praise shall continually be in mouth" (Psalm 34:1). By making a declaration to bless the Lord at all times, it is virtually impossible to live in any form of defeat. Your protection is that you have decided to walk with God in your praise through each day, no matter what happens or comes your way.

DAY 1: THANKSGIVING

Promise: *Seven times a day do I praise thee, because of thy righteous judgment. Great peace have they which love thy law: and nothing shall offend them (Psalm 119: 165).*

Practice: A daily focus on the goodness of God in our lives brings forth an attitude of gratitude and thanksgiving. While praising God seven times a day may seem a bit much, such praise is dwarfed in comparison to the constant grace, mercy, protection and provision we have all day long. We eagerly jump in and out of our vehicles, frustrated by any small delay in traffic and drive fifty-five miles per hour or more on multi-lane highways, only inches away from other drivers, and still we arrive at our destinations safely.

We rush in and out of the grocery store purchasing whatever we need and most of what we want, showing great disdain if we have to wait behind one or two people in line.

There are blessings occurring twenty-four hours a day, seven days a week, but they are often clouded by the price of small inconveniences. The smallest inconvenience offends us and disturbs our peace. We are offended by what we hear on the news or see on television, we are offended by what a family member or friend did or did not do, we are offended if our names are not called or we are not acknowledged for our contributions. Often, if you really think about it, being offended by every little thing is a copout, a way to gain the compassion from those around us.

Practice praise and worship and adoration of God. Look to Him for strength and resolution of your major issues. Do all that you do to glorify God, and allow Him to reward you in His own way. Today, meditate on the word and laws of God and you will find *great* peace and *nothing* said or done throughout the day should offend you.

Prayer: Lord, fill me with an attitude of thanksgiving and gratitude. Help me to search out and find you in even what I perceive to be inconveniences in my life. Teach me to count my blessings and learn to praise you for each one. I thank you for granting me the peace to practice patience. Allow it to have its perfect work in my life. Lord, your Word says that we should not be overcome with evil, but overcome evil with good (Romans 12:21). Help me, Lord, to embrace your peace, meditate on your word, and bless your name at all times so that nothing that I face today shall offend me. Amen.

Psalm 100:4: *"Enter into His gates with thanksgiving, and into His gates with praise: Be thankful unto Him, and bless His name."*

Physical Activity:

1. Warm-up
2. Stretch
3. Workout Card: Day 1

EXERCISE: DAY 1	BEGINNER	MODERATE	ADVANCED
Cardio	#1 x 15 minutes	#2 x 10 minutes	#3 x 7 minutes
Leg Work #1	10 times	15 times	20 times
Arm Work #1 & 2	10 times	15 times	20 times
Ab Work #1 & 2	10 times	15 times	20 times
Ball Work #1 & 2	10 times	15 times	20 times

DAY 2 : CRYING OUT

Promise: *The whole multitude of the disciples began to rejoice and praise God with a loud voice for all the mighty works that they had seen … And some of the Pharisees from among the multitude said unto him, "Master, rebuke thy disciples" And He [Jesus] answered and said unto them, "I tell you that, if these should hold their peace, the stones would immediately cry out"* (Luke 19:37-40).

Practice: We have seen God do some mighty works in our lives and in the lives of those around us. He has earned our praise, and He is truly worthy of it. God will get His praise even if He has to take the example of a lifeless, limbless, motionless stone and give it a mouth to praise Him. This is a display of how important praise and worship is to God. He did not use an animal with eyes, ears, a nose, and a mouth to replace our praise. He used a stone. Considering all of the physical blessings you have—sight, hearing, walking, talking, thinking, building, and even loving—would you let a stone steal your praise?

You were obviously thought of much higher than a stone, but Jesus uses this lower level of creation to express the necessity of praise. Praise God! It is He who has made you and given you all that you have and made you all that you are. Do not allow a stone to cry out in your place! Praise God! He is worthy of all your praise.

There are some people who believe it does not take extremes or loud vocal expressions to praise God. The scriptures disagree. The Psalmist mandates that we make a joyful "noise" unto the Lord. Jesus clearly states in the text that the stones will "cry out." This does not seem at all silent to me. Only you know what God has done for you. Only you can give Him glory from your heart. Let us go forth today in praise and worship. Today, speak to yourself in psalms and hymns and spiritual songs, singing and making melody in your heart to the Lord; giving thanks always for all things unto God and the Father in the name of our Lord Jesus Christ (Ephesians 5:19-20).

Prayer: Lord God, help me not to be ashamed of the Gospel of Jesus Christ. I pray for boldness to glorify your name in word and deed. Help me to know and understand that I am fearfully and wonderfully made in the image of God. I pray for Holy Ghost boldness to praise you in good times and in challenging times. Lord, grant me a praying and praising spirit. Lord, you are worthy to receive honor and power and glory. The angels bow before you. They worship and adore you. You are the King of kings and the Lord of lords, and I will not withhold your praise. I thank you for the wonderful things that you have done in my life. I praise you for life, health, and strength. Amen. "Blessed be the King that cometh in the Name of the Lord: Peace in Heaven, and Glory in the Highest" (Luke 19:38).

Psalm 150: *"Praise ye the Lord. Praise God in his sanctuary: praise him in the firmament of his power. Praise him for his mighty acts: praise him according to his excellent greatness. Praise him with the sound of the trumpet: praise him with the psaltery and harp. Praise him with the timbrel and dance: praise him with the stringed instrument and organs. Praise him upon the loud cymbals: praise him upon the high sounding cymbals. Let everything that hath breath praise the Lord. Praise ye the Lord."*

Physical Activity:

1. Warm-up
2. Stretch
3. Workout Card: Day 2

EXERCISE: DAY 2	BEGINNER	MODERATE	ADVANCED
Cardio #5	10 minutes	15 minutes	20 minutes
Leg Work #2	10 times	15 times	20 times
Arm Work #3 & 4	10 times	15 times	20 times
Ab Work #2 & 3	10 times	15 times	20 times
Ball Work #1 & 3	10 times	15 times	20 times

DAY 3: PRAISE BIRTHD FROM GRIEF

Promise: *"And she was in bitterness of soul, and prayed unto the LORD, and wept sore. And she vowed a vow, and said, O LORD of hosts, if thou wilt indeed look on the affliction of thine handmaid, and remember me, and not forget thine handmaid, but wilt give unto thine handmaid a man child, then I will give him unto the LORD all the days of his life, and there shall no razor come upon his head. And they rose up in the morning early, and worshipped before the LORD, and returned, and came to their house to Ramah: and Elkanah knew Hannah his wife; and the LORD remembered her"* (1 Samuel 1:10-11 and 19).

Practice: Hannah was a woman well-favored and provided for by her husband, yet she was stricken with great grief because she could not have children. Her husband's other wife tormented and mocked her because of this. Then Hannah remembered the house of the Lord. Hannah not only cried out to the Lord, but she made a vow to give the first fruit of her womb back to God. God honored Hannah's plea, promise, and praise. He gave her a son.

In 1 Samuel Chapter 2, Hannah's mourning is turned into gladness. What is the source of your grief? What is making you unhappy? Is there one thing that you cannot seem to achieve, no matter what you do? Jesus is the answer! I am convinced that it is the anointing oil of the Holy Spirit of God that breaks depression and sadness from our hearts. God wants us blessed with every good and perfect gift. No good thing will He withhold from them that walk uprightly (Psalm 84:11). If you have not gotten the good desires of your heart, it is because of one of the following: 1) God desires your devotion. 2) You are not ready for it. 3) It is not good for you. Every good and perfect gift comes from God. The blessings of the Lord make us rich and add no sorrow. Today, add fasting and praise to your prayers and petitions to God, and watch Him do for you what He did for Hannah in her time of grief.

Prayer: Father God, heal my heart and my mind. Fill the deep-rooted voids that have disappointed me and caused me to be embittered, unhappy, and ungrateful. Father, I offer to you my garment of grief and heaviness, and I ask you to give me a new garment of praise, thanksgiving, and contentment. I love you, Lord, and I know that you love me. Teach me to love and pass through my pain so that you may be glorified in my life. Let your light shine brightly through me. I thank you even now, Lord, for filling me with your Holy Spirit. I pray that my desires may line up with your will for my life. Hallelujah! Amen!

Psalm 127: *"Except the LORD build the house, they labour in vain that build it: except the LORD keep the city, the watchman waketh but in vain. It is vain for you to rise up early, to sit up late, to eat the bread of sorrows: for so he giveth his beloved sleep. Lo, children are an heritage of the LORD: and the fruit of the womb is his reward. As arrows are in the hand of a mighty man; so are children of the youth. Happy is the man that hath his quiver full of them: they shall not be ashamed, but they shall speak with the enemies in the gate."*

Physical Activity:
1. Warm-up
2. Stretch
3. Workout Card: Day 3

EXERCISE: DAY 3	BEGINNER	MODERATE	ADVANCED
Cardio	#1 x 16 minutes	#2 x 11 minutes	#3 x 8 minutes
Leg Work #3	10 times	15 times	20 times
Arm Work #5	10 times	15 times	20 times
Ab Work #4 & 5	10 times	15 times	20 times
Ball Work #1 & 4	10 times	15 times	20 times

DAY 4: EARTHQUAKE PRAISE

Promise: *"And at midnight Paul and Silas prayed, and sang praises unto God: and the prisoners heard them. And suddenly there was a great earthquake, so that the foundations of the prison were shaken: and immediately all the doors were opened, and every one's bands were loosed"* (Acts 16:25-26).

Practice: After being mocked by a girl with a spirit of divination for many days, Paul, along with Silas, turned and rebuked the spirit and commanded that it come out of the girl. This girl was being prostituted by this spirit to bring her masters a lot of money. When the power of the spirit left the girl and they lost their gain, they then accused Paul and Silas of being lawless troublemakers. Paul and Silas were thrown into jail for standing up for the gospel. Without wrath or doubting, or any form of resentment, Paul and Silas both prayed and sang praises to God. They sang and prayed so loudly that the prisoners heard them.

God honors prayer combined with praise. He sent forth an earthquake that not only loosed Paul and Silas, but everyone in the prison, including the guard who, as a result, gave his life to Christ.

Praise and worship has to explode past the sanctuary at the local church. We must be trained to pray and praise God in the midnight hour so that we can make it to the morning light. Some of the challenges that we face, which seem unjust, may not have anything to do with us. Often, we are sent into jungles and prisons just so that others may learn and see how Christians respond to God in trying times. We must not withhold our prayers and praises to God because of the place that we are in or because of who is around us. If only one person's heavy burden is lifted, if only one soul is saved, if only one person is delivered, then your prayer and praise is not in vain.

Let us go forth today and produce earthshaking praises unto our God. He is so worthy. He has blessed us to be a blessing. We praise God not because we are exempt from the trials and tribulations of life, but because, with Him in the middle, we can expect a favorable outcome for ourselves and for those around us. In the jungle, melodies and praise were my way of staying covered and motivated during my stay. In only a few days, I realized that the melodies and praise blessed my entire tribe.

Prayer: Father God, I pray for bold faith, a faith that is strong enough to praise you in the middle of my storm and expect you to show up and shine on my situation. Help me, oh Lord, to continue to praise you when I pray to fully engage your answer to my dilemma. Lord, please bless my unbelief so that I will not be ashamed of the Gospel of Jesus Christ. Use me, heavenly Father, as a vessel of prayer and worship that will draw people to your loving-kindness so, like the prison guard, they will ask, "What must I do to be saved?" Father, I pray for my friends and family who are imprisoned by many burdens, habits, and challenges. Help me to remember that this Christian walk is not all about me, though it includes me. Shape me into a powerhouse of faith that can be used to deliver others through earthquaking prayer and praise.

Psalm 40: 1-3: *I waited patiently for the LORD; and He inclined unto me, and heard my cry. He brought me up also out of an horrible pit, out of the miry clay, and set my foot upon a* *rock, and established my goings. And He hath put a new song in my mouth, even praise unto our God: many shall see it, and fear, and shall trust in the LORD.*

Physical Activity:
1. Warm-up
2. Stretch
3. Workout Card: Day 4

EXERCISE: DAY 4	BEGINNER	MODERATE	ADVANCED
Cardio #4	set of 25 non-stop	7 minutes	10 minutes
Leg Work #4	10 times	15 times	20 times
Arm Work #1 & 2	10 times	15 times	20 times
Ab Work #3 & 4	10 times	15 times	20 times
Ball Work #1 & 5	10 times	15 times	20 times

DAY 5: RESTORATION

Promise: *"And I will restore to you the years that the locust hath eaten, the cankerworm, and the caterpiller, and the palmerworm, my great army which I sent among you.*

And ye shall eat in plenty, and be satisfied, and praise the name of the LORD your God, that hath dealt wondrously with you: and my people shall never be ashamed" (Joel 2:25-26).

Practice: Sometimes your faith and hope in God can keep you in a place or situation long after you have exhausted all of your energy, love, hopes, and dreams. You have given your all and you have nothing left, but your faith keeps you there because you know that God is able. Although your storage is empty and most of the zeal and energy you had for the faith is depleted, somehow when you wake you still have expectation through God's blessed assurance. That is called faith. Without faith, it is impossible to please God. The name Joel means "Yahweh is God." As sure as God is God, He has not forgotten your faithfulness, your diligence, and your labor of love. The scriptures instruct us to pray for those who hate us and despitefully use us and speak all manner of evil against us. We are instructed to bless and not curse those who cause us great pain. Praying in pain is what I call it. Much of the time, the people who fall into this category of "those who hate you and despitefully use you and speak all matter of evil against you" are the people closest to you.

God is God, and He has promised through the prophet Joel to restore what seems to be the impossible. God promises to restore what has already been consumed, digested, and processed as waste. He promises to restore what has been depleted, emptied, and completely used up. The years that have been consumed and distributed in the flesh of thousands of locusts and hundreds of these four specific worms, is virtually impossible for our minds to conceive. Joel tapped into this realm of carnal impossibility to ensure us that God is capable of restoring everything that has been consumed. Perhaps it is your marriage, your joy, a pursuit of a higher education, peace within your household, or reconciliation of lost loved ones. No matter what it is, God can and will restore what you have lost.

Yahweh is God, and there is nothing too hard for Him. Before I entered into the jungle and found those pineapples, I had already suffered tremendous loss. Several years earlier, I experienced a painful, yet necessary, divorce. I had recently lost my greatest support and confidant, my mother, to a sudden death. My greatest challenge was leaving the familiarity of a community life I had built over a decade. It has not been easy, but it has been worth it. God has replenished my life with great counsel, community, and contentment. The most important part of restoration is learning to "rest" and know that "Yahweh is God."

Prayer: Father God, my storage is empty. I need to be restored. I bring my emptiness to you. I bring my brokenness to you. I bring my loneliness to you. I am coming to you because I have labored in love and I am heavily laden, and now I need rest. I thank you, Lord, that when I rest in you I am both replenished and refreshed, and I am totally restored. Shape me, make me, and revive me, Lord Jesus. I have experienced tragic events and spiritual setbacks, but I ask you LORD to make me over in the spirit. Make me faster, stronger, and better than I have ever been. Make me a new creature in Christ so that I can move past what I lost and what was stolen from me. Lord, I thank you for making me to eat in plenty, being totally satisfied so that I may praise your Holy name. Hallelujah!

Psalm 91:15-16: *"He shall call upon me, and I will answer Him: I will be with Him in trouble; I will deliver Him, and honor Him. With long life will I satisfy Him, and show Him my salvation."*

Physical Activity:
1. Warm-up
2. Stretch
3. Workout Card: Day 5

EXERCISE: DAY 5	BEGINNER	MODERATE	ADVANCED
Cardio	#1 x 17 minutes	#2 x 12 minutes	#3 x 9 minutes
Leg Work #5	10 times	15 times	20 times
Arm Work #3 & 4	10 times	15 times	20 times
Ab Work #5 & 1	10 times	15 times	20 times
Ball Work #1 & 2	10 times	15 times	20 times

DAY 6: "YET PRAISE"

Promise: *"Although the fig tree shall not blossom, neither shall fruit be in the vines; the labour of the olive shall fail, and the fields shall yield no meat; the flock shall be cut off from the fold, and there shall be no herd in the stalls: Yet I will rejoice in the LORD, I will joy in the God of my salvation. The LORD God is my strength, and he will make my feet like hinds' feet, and he will make me to walk upon mine high places…"* (Habakkuk 3:17-19).

Practice: Habakkuk shows us the highest level of praise in this scripture. A "Yet Praise" is described as the praise that does not produce any fruit. It is the praise that is made when your bank account is in the negative. It is the praise that is made when your best friend betrays you. It is a praise that is made when your children run away from home or become progressively disobedient. It is a praise that is made when you have to say good-bye to a loved one. Only mature Christians who understand that God is to be glorified and magnified at all times have a "yet praise." Out of frustration with wickedness and the oppression of the weak, Habakkuk turns to God, questioning His passive attention to the ills of the world. God assures the prophet that He is large and in charge and that, in an appointed time, the vision that was being revealed to Habakkuk would speak and not lie. God admonished Habakkuk to wait for the vision, for though it tarried, it would come to pass. (Habakkuk 2:2-3: *"And the LORD answered me, and said, Write the vision, and make it plain upon tables, that he may run that readeth it. For the vision is yet for an appointed time, but at the end it shall speak, and not lie: though it tarry, wait for it; because it will surely come, it will not tarry."*)

Be encouraged, my brothers and my sisters, and know that the righteous must live in complete devotion and faithfulness to God, no matter what. There are many instances in the Bible where it seemed like the vision would not come to pass. Dozens of scriptures reference God's chosen people on the brink of destruction when God stepped in to deliver.

Do you have a yet praise? In order to get through the darkest night, you will need a yet praise. To get through seasons of spiritual famine and drought, you will need a yet praise. On multiple occasions, I found myself in a position of yet praise. In seasons like these, we must activate the combined power of the promises of God with praise and worship.

The Achilles tendon is the strongest tendon in the body. You use it when you run, jump, bounce, and walk with a decent stride. Last spring, while playing basketball with a family member, I suffered a partial tear in my Achilles tendon. While it was painful, swollen, black and blue, I could still get around and did not need surgery. Fitness is my profession, and many spectators at the gym were shocked to see me "yet" come to the gym to complete modified workouts with a prescribed boot on my leg and a smile on my face.

As inconvenient as this injury may have been, I was aware of my flawless track record, so I worshipped God. In high school, I leaped the hundred meter hurdles and played four years of basketball without one injury. In college, I was a standout basketball player who often plunged into the stands and clock tables after loose balls without injury. For decades, I have bounced around performing many athletic feats, even living in one of the greatest jungles in the world. God has provided me with a lifetime of blessings and excellent health. I praise Him even in temporary seasons of inconvenience. Hallelujah! Put a yet praise on your lips even in your grim situations. God is worthy and waiting to prove that to you!

Prayer: Hallelujah, Oh Glory! Hallelujah! Amen! Lord, I praise you because you have been so very good to me. I will retain the memories of good times and blessings to take me through seasons of trials and tribulations. You are a good God and a stronghold in the day of trouble, in the day of famine, and in the day of desolation. Your Word assures me that the name of the Lord is a strong tower to which the righteous run and are safe. Thank you, Lord, for being my strong tower. I pray for a yet praise. I praise that it is strengthened with each season. I offer praise to you, oh Lord, in the midst of my storm. As I walk through the valley of the shadow of death, I will fear no evil because you are with me. Teach me to know without doubt that you are still Jehovah Jireh, the God who provides, even when all of my storehouses are empty and the work I do produces no fruit. Yet will I praise you Lord, for you have done great and mighty things. This season shall pass and you will make my feet like the feet of deer and set me up for great and mighty things to come. Hallelujah!

Psalm 77:10-14: *"And I said, this is my infirmity: but I will remember the years of the right hand of the Most High. I will remember the works of the LORD: surely I will remember thy wonders of old. I will meditate also of all thy work, and talk of thy doings. Thy way, O God, is in the sanctuary: who is so great a God as our God? Thou art the God that doest wonders: thou hast declared thy strength among the people."*

Physical Activity:

1. Warm-up
2. Stretch
3. Workout Card: Day 6

EXERCISE: DAY 6	BEGINNER	MODERATE	ADVANCED
Cardio #4	25 non-stop	7 minutes	10 minutes
Cardio #5	10 minutes	15 minutes	20 minutes
Leg Work #1	10 times	15 times	20 times
Arm Work #5	10 times	15 times	20 times
Ab Work #1 & 2	10 times	15 times	20 times
Ball Work #1 & 3	10 times	15 times	20 times

DAY 7: HALLELUJAH! OH GLORY! HALLELUJAH! AMEN!

Promise: *"And a second time they said, "Hallelujah! HER SMOKE RISES UP FOREVER AND EVER." And the twenty-four elders and the four living creatures fell down and worshiped God who sits on the throne saying, "Amen. Hallelujah!" And a voice came from the throne, saying, "Give praise to our God, all you His bond-servants, you who fear Him, the small and the great." Then I heard something like the voice of a great multitude and like the sound of many waters and like the sound of mighty peals of thunder, saying, "Hallelujah! For the Lord our God, the Almighty, reigns"* (Revelation 19:3-6, NASB).

Practice: I only recently learned of the above passage in the Book of the Revelation after being labeled the "Hallelujah Lady" because of my radical praise of "Hallelujah, Oh Glory... Hallelujah, Amen" in the Amazon and on the CBS Early Show. I had no idea that this chapter is referred to as the Fourfold Hallelujah. Obviously, Hallelujah is so delightful to God that it is repeated not twice, not three times, but four times. Initially, "Hallelujah Oh Glory" was birthed out of my heart as a way of glorifying God for the mighty acts and wonders He performed in my life. While I did not know of this scriptural reference, I did know that this level of worship felt right and took me to higher spiritual levels. I also learned that those subjected to the barrack-style praise felt great peace and freedom.

The world is rapidly changing, and with this change morality is becoming as obsolete as VCRs and landline telephones. I am not certain of how it will all turn out, but I do know that God will be glorified on Earth. Hallelujah is the highest praise, and Revelation teaches us that it a prerequisite to a position around the throne of God. Hallelujah is a congregation or community command to engage in worship of the Most High God. If you plan to see God, just remember that, based on this text, He requires praise and adoration. Why not practice worshiping God right now while you are still here? His blessings follow praise and obedience both here and now as well as in the heavens. May the Lord be magnified and glorified forever!

Prayer: Thank you, Lord, for seven days of praise! Hallelujah! I thank you Lord for insight and wisdom. I thank you for your mercy and your grace. Lord, fill me with a praying and praising spirit so that when I get to Heaven, I can fit right in. Lord, I worship you for what you have done in my life, for what you are doing in my life, and for who you are in my life. Lord, I praise you for the good times and the bad. I praise you when I am happy and when I am sad. Lord, I praise you because you are good. I thank you for your yes and I thank you for your no. I thank you when I win and I thank you when I lose. I thank you, Lord, for all things. I thank you for Jesus Christ. I thank you, Lord Jesus, for being my personal savior and advocate, the link between God and me. It is because of you and your loyal obedience that I can tug on the heartstrings of God with praise and feel His Holy Spirit move through me and on my behalf. Hallelujah to your name, oh God! You are worthy, and I will not let a stone "out-cry" me. Amen!

Psalm 113: *"Praise ye the LORD. Praise, O ye servants of the LORD, praise the name of the LORD. Blessed be the name of the LORD from this time forth and for evermore. From the rising of the sun unto the going down of the same the LORD's* *name is to be praised. The LORD is high above all nations, and his glory above the heavens. Who is like unto the LORD our God, who dwelleth on high, Who humbleth himself to behold the things that are in heaven, and in the earth! He raiseth up the poor out of the dust, and lifteth the needy out of the dunghill; That he may set him with princes, even with the princes of his people. He maketh the barren woman to keep house, and to be a joyful mother of children. Praise ye the LORD."*

Physical Activity:

1. Warm-up
2. Stretch
3. Workout Card: Day 7 – Rest!

EXERCISE: DAY 7	BEGINNER	MODERATE	ADVANCED
	REST	REST	REST

Day 7: Remember the Sabbath day and to keep it holy, and God will remember you. God rested on the seventh day, and so should you!

Week 2

Fruit of the Spirit

The fruit of the spirit is a major "peace" of the pineapple. It is through the Holy Spirit, the Spirit of Truth, that God is omnipresent, moving and operating in our lives. The fruit of the spirit is strategically organized in Galatians 5:22-23. The first of the fruits is *love*. For without a foundation based on agape, self-emptying love, all else will fail. Love won the victory at Calvary—not power or might, just love. God so loved the entire world that He gave His only begotten son Jesus Christ to be crucified, buried, and resurrected on the third day for all of our sins. Abraham's faithfulness and obedience to God in the attempted sacrifice of his only son, Isaac, was a precursor to God's actual sacrifice of His only begotten son, Jesus Christ. Now that is love. Love conquers all. Love is the base of spiritual fruit.

Joy and peace are next because they are byproducts of love. Joy is calmness and a walk of divine, blessed assurance that the world cannot give and thus cannot take away. Peace, listed third among the fruits of the spirit, is derived from the word *eirene,* which means health, prosperity, quietness, and rest. This is a much needed healthy spiritual snack in a fast-paced world powered by demands and stress. Joy and peace are followed by longsuffering. Longsuffering, just as it states, is the ability to suffer long. It is having a high tolerance and endurance for what is uncomfortable. It is actually very painful, but this suffering is not in vain. Through it, character, integrity, courage, and humility are birthed. These virtues are produced through patience.

The next fruit on the list is gentleness. This gentleness is not that of a baby's skin, a rose petal, or even soft speech. In this context, gentleness means moral excellence. *Chrestotes*, another word for gentleness, also means excellence in character or demeanor. We could all use a little more *chrestotes* in our personae.

The expression of goodness is another manifestation of the Spirit. Goodness is not only the premise of being good, but of committing good acts. Beneficence is another word for goodness, which means virtue. It is further defined as a willingness to help others. Could you imagine how much better your day would be if it was filled with more beneficence?

Faith is the tie that binds the fruit of the spirit and keeps it all together. As the seventh place holder, faith is the entire reason for our being, for staying, hoping, and growing. The ultimate warfare is never about the trial or the attack. The warfare is to either test or take your faith.

Meekness is accomplished when pride is diminished. This meekness makes us confident and filled with the compassion of Christ without a hint of arrogance. The divine line of the spiritual vine is completed with temperance or self-control. Self-control is the greatest personal power one can master. Temperance must be executed to complete even the smallest task. You must use temperance to complete your six-day workout regiment. You need temperance to be faithful to an unfaithful spouse. You need temperance to remain celibate in your singleness. You need temperance when it comes to studying God's word, fasting, and praying. Temperance, or self-control, is the engine of our souls. Many people have great faith, a command of God's Word, or even a religious system, but lack the self-control that is needed to draw near to God and follow through with the tasks and commands He gives us.

The greatest and most dynamic benefit to walking a spirit-filled and spirit-led life is becoming a new creature in Jesus Christ. There is no need to ponder the things, habits, and people of your past. There is no need to harbor unforgiveness and bitterness toward past and present abusers. Let not your heart be troubled or shameful about the unsettling facts of your genealogy. The fruit of the spirit is the nature and character of God almighty. In choosing to embrace the fruit of the spirit of God, we embrace the character of God, thereby rejecting all else. We do not have to take on the sinful nature of our earthly fathers, for we can walk in newness of life through spiritual adoption of the nature of God, our heavenly Father.

DAY 1: LOVE

Promise: *"Beloved, let us love one another: for love is of God; and every one that loveth is born of God, and knoweth God. He that loveth not knoweth not God; for God is love. In this was manifested the love of God toward us, because that God sent his only begotten Son into the world, that we might live through him. Herein is love, not that we loved God, but that he loved us, and sent his Son to be the propitiation for our sins. Beloved, if God so loved us, we ought also to love one another"* (1 John 4:7-11).

Practice: The first fruit of the spirit is love. This love is not one that is stimulated by attractiveness or desire for affection. This love is expressed unconditionally. This love pre-exists us, our motives, or intentions. This love is to be likened to that of parents toward their unborn babies. For nine months, a baby is unaware of the care, attention, and preparation made for its arrival. Once the baby is born, it is still unaware of all of the love around it, and it only has one motive: to express need. God loves us the same way. If you look back over your life, you can see God's loving hands all over it. He has changed some messy situations for you. He has constantly fed you when you were physically and spiritually hungry. He has protected you from the consequences of your own bad choices. A child "learns" to love her parents although she could never fully reciprocate that love. As a Christian, think of it this way: God first loved us and this love can only be reciprocated through us loving our fellow man. I always wondered how God loves those who hate Him and blaspheme His name. I am talking about those who outwardly denounce Jesus Christ and embrace satan. After meditating on this question for many days, God took me to

Genesis 2:7: *"And the Lord God formed man of the dust of the ground, and breathed into his nostrils the breath of life; and man became a living soul."*

Every person upon this earth that has breath, the good, the bad, and even the wickedly ugly, has acquired breath, which is a form of spirit, from Adam. Adam acquired this breath of life from God himself, and thus a piece of God is in each of us. Each time a soul does not return to God, He is grieved, for He has lost a part of himself. Therefore, it is vital that we share the good news with every living soul so that they may return to the Father. As simple as this may seem, Jesus gives His disciples a specific outline in how to go about sharing the gospel: *"Behold, I send you forth as sheep in the midst of wolves: be ye therefore wise as serpents, and harmless as doves"* (Matthew 10:16).

Because of past hurts and rejection, we have withdrawn from sharing the gospel of Jesus Christ and the love of God with others, especially with those we find unresponsive, resistant, and downright disrespectful. Our challenge today is to implement wisdom in our attempt to both love and share the Gospel of Jesus Christ. Expressed unconditional, self-emptying love can only be found in God and in our accepting this love from Him. Only then can we begin to love God through expressing love toward our fellow man. God is love.

Prayer: Father God, thank you for your loving-kindness toward me. Thank you for loving me through my sins and past my faults. How understanding and merciful you have been to me. I thank you for the ultimate expression of love, your son Jesus Christ. Thank you, Lord Jesus, for your demonstration of love through the laying down of your life that I might live through you. Teach me to love my neighbor as I love myself. As I remember your pressing love for me when I was yet lost in sin, fill me with the wisdom and compassion to love others through their present plights. I love you, Lord. Help me to honor you by allowing the love of the Holy Spirit to live and move and breathe through me each day. This is my prayer today, oh Lord, that you would teach me to really love others.

Psalm 18:1-3: *"I will love thee, O LORD, my strength. The LORD is my rock, and my fortress, and my deliverer; my God, my strength, in whom I will trust; my buckler, and the horn of my salvation, and my high tower. I will call upon the LORD, who is worthy to be praised: so shall I be saved from mine enemies."*

Physical Activity:
1. Warm-up
2. Stretch
3. Workout Card: Day 1 – Workout Phase 2

EXERCISE: DAY 1	BEGINNER	MODERATE	ADVANCED
Cardio	#1 x 18 minutes	#2 x 13 minutes	#3 x 10 minutes
Leg Work #2	2 x 10 times	2 x 15 times	2 x 20 times
Arm Work #1 & 2	2 x 10 times	2 x 15 times	2 x 20 times
Ab Work #1 & 2	2 x 10 times	2 x 15 times	2 x 20 times
Ball Work #1 & 2	2 x 10 times	2 x 15 times	2 x 20 times

DAY 2: JOY AND PEACE

Promise: *"Let not then your good be evil spoken of: For the Kingdom of God is not meat and drink; but righteousness, and peace, and joy in the Holy Ghost"* (Romans 14:17).

Practice: How pleasant it is to be in the presence of those filled with joy. Joy is not restricted to laughter or pleasant circumstances. Joy is a state of mind. It is a blessed assurance that produces enduring and sacred peace. Joy and peace go hand-in-hand, because you cannot have joy and no peace or have peace and no joy. This dual spiritual fruit is the mainstay of the Christian diet. The adversary of the human soul is constantly attempting to confuse our balanced diet with junk food. Have you ever witnessed a Christian of great faith with diligence to the ministry suffer what seemed to be unnecessary or unwarranted difficulties, and yet the person was filled with joy and peace? These mature Christians have their souls anchored to the Lord Jesus Christ so that the storms and harsh winds of life may rock them, but they shall not be moved.

Jesus leaves us with this assurance: *"And ye now therefore have sorrow: but I will see you again, and your heart shall rejoice, and your joy no man taketh from you"* (John 16:22). And, in John 14:27, He leaves us with divine peace: *"Peace I leave with you, my peace I give unto you: not as the world giveth, give I unto you. Let not your heart be troubled, neither let it be afraid."* Clearly, Jesus indicates in these scriptures that the joy and peace He freely gives us do not come from the world and the world cannot take them away. Thank God! Could you imagine having your joy revoked or your peace repossessed? That would be tragic. In departing this life, Jesus knew the weaknesses and doubts of His followers. He encouraged them not to let their hearts be troubled or afraid. His followers, much like those of us today, were allowing themselves to become agitated, disturbed, intimidated, cowardly, and unsettled.

In the game of football, the team is led by the quarterback. The quarterback is protected by big offensive linemen so that he can make clear decisions about moving the entire team down the field and past the defense. The protection this line provides is called "the pocket." If the quarterback remains in the pocket, he is safe. However, if the pocket breaks down, he becomes unsettled and he must scramble, risking the possibility of getting "sacked." In the Christian's life, joy and peace are the offensive line of the spirit. Abiding in the joy and peace of Jesus Christ will protect us from the spiritual blows and sacks of life. Today, let us manifest the joy and peace of the spirit that Jesus has promised us. Let us determine today that no matter what comes our way, we will abide in that joy and peace, and it shall abide in us. Greater is the joy and peace of God operating in and through us than that of the world. The world did not give it, so do not allow the troubles of the world to take it away. Whoever "they" are, they did not give you joy and peace either, so do not let "them" take it away, not another day, ever again.

Prayer: Lord, make me hear joy and gladness. Fill me with a peace that surpasses all understanding. Lord, I pray for the stability of your mercy and grace so that I may abide in your love and peace. Let your love and peace abide in me. Father, let not my heart be troubled about the changes and challenges I face in life. Help me to daily consume the fruits of joy and peace that my spirit might be well-balanced and whole. Lord, I want to walk in the essence of your joy and peace from this day forward and forevermore. Lord, grant me the serenity to accept the things that I cannot change, the courage and strength to change the things that I can, and the wisdom to know the difference between what I can and cannot change.* Thank you, Lord, for all is well with me and my soul.

Psalm 51:10-13: *"Create in me a clean heart, O God; and renew a right spirit within me. Cast me not away from thy presence; and take not thy holy spirit from me. Restore unto me the joy of thy salvation; and uphold me with thy free spirit. Then will I teach transgressors thy ways; and sinners shall be converted unto thee."*

Psalm 37:37: *"Mark the perfect man, and behold the upright: for the end of that man is peace."*

Physical Activity:
1. Warm-up
2. Stretch
3. Workout Card: Day 2 – Workout Phase 2

EXERCISE: DAY 2	BEGINNER	MODERATE	ADVANCED
Cardio #5	12 minutes	17 minutes	22 minutes
Leg Work #2	2 x 10 times	2 x 15 times	2 x 20 times
Arm Work #3 & 4	2 x 10 times	2 x 15 times	2 x 20 times
Ab Work #2 & 3	2 x 10 times	2 x 15 times	2 x 20 times
Ball Work #1 & 3	2 x 10 times	2 x 15 times	2 x 20 times

* "The Serenity Prayer" by Reinhold Niebuhr.

DAY 3: LONGSUFFERING

Promise: *"Giving no offence in any thing, that the ministry be not blamed: But in all things approving ourselves as the ministers of God, in much patience, in afflictions, in necessities, in distresses, In stripes, in imprisonments, in tumults, in labours, in watchings, in fastings; By pureness, by knowledge, by longsuffering, by kindness, by the Holy Ghost, by love unfeigned, By the word of truth, by the power of God, by the armour of righteousness on the right hand and on the left, By honour and dishonour, by evil report and good report: as deceivers, and yet true; as unknown, and yet well known; as dying, and, behold, we live; as chastened, and not killed; As sorrowful, yet always rejoicing; as poor, yet making many rich; as having nothing, and yet possessing all things"* (2 Corinthians 6:3-10).

Practice: Longsuffering is one of the fruits of the spirit that is a bitter piece to swallow. The acquisition process is not only uncomfortable, but very long and tiring. Because the Holy Spirit comes from God, we can search the scriptures and find that God himself initiates the first demonstration of all of the spiritual fruits. His longsuffering tolerance of our disobedience and rebellion is exclaimed by Him as early as Exodus 34:6, as He passes in front of an outdone Moses to restore the first set of tablets that were broken: *"And the LORD passed by before him, and proclaimed, The LORD, The LORD God, merciful and gracious, longsuffering, and abundant in goodness and truth, Keeping mercy for thousands, forgiving iniquity and transgression and sin, and that will by no means clear the guilty; visiting the iniquity of the fathers upon the children, and upon the children's children, unto the third and to the fourth generation."* Amazingly, God proclaims that there is a distinct difference between His mercy and His wrath. For thousands of generations, God's grace and mercy follow those who love Him, but the visitation of the iniquity of the fathers upon the children and children's children only extends to the third and fourth generations. Thank God that He executes longsuffering on our behalf so that our children are not bound in iniquity for our selfish faults.

On the other hand, if man were to decide the fate of his enemies and those who hate him, he would visit iniquity upon his enemy unto the thousandth generation and maybe show mercy and kindness toward four generations of those who love him. God is demonstrating His tolerance, patience, and forgiveness on our behalf. This is why He can make the sun shine on the just and the unjust. He transfers traits to us through the fruit of the spirit. Though they are slowly absorbed, others may never see God's grace and mercy without our demonstration of longsuffering. Others may never be redeemed and set free if we fail to be longsuffering in love, peace, and joy. Choose forgiveness in longsuffering. Pray for strength to finish the course. We must not run from the discomforts of longsuffering, thereby aborting a major portion of our spiritual growth and development. God knows how much suffering we can handle. Let us approach today, not in despair or disdain of our longsuffering, but with a renewed hope and expectation that we will be new creatures when the patience is complete.

Prayer: Father God, I want to be made whole and complete. I want to lack nothing. I want to be everything you have created me to be. I realize that longsuffering may very well be part of that process, so I am submitting my will to you. Transform me, shape me, make me, and guide me until I look just like you. Toughen me with more tolerance and patience for the long road ahead. Pack my spirit with the fresh fruits of your love, peace, and joy. I am ready to go through this process, oh Lord. I only ask that you manifest yourself and walk with me. I cannot do this alone. I have become weary. I thank you for your Word in Isaiah that states that even the youth shall faint and be weary, the young men shall utterly fall, but they that wait upon the Lord shall renew their strength; they shall mount up with wings as eagles; they shall run and not be weary; they shall walk and not faint. Your Word also encourages me to be not weary in well doing for I shall reap if I faint not. Lord, I am weary. Help me to hold on until you are finished with this season in my life, or until you deliver me. Lord, as I wait upon you, teach me to renew my strength, to run without being tired, and let me walk without fainting. In the name of Jesus Christ, none of this longsuffering is ever in vain.

Psalm 90:12-17: *"So teach us to number our days, that we may apply our hearts unto wisdom. Return, O LORD, how long? and let it repent thee concerning thy servants. O satisfy us early with thy mercy; that we may rejoice and be glad all our days. Make us glad according to the days wherein thou hast afflicted us, and the years wherein we have seen evil. Let thy work appear unto thy servants, and thy glory unto their children. And let the beauty of the LORD our God be upon us: and establish thou the work of our hands upon us; yea, the work of our hands establish thou it."*

Physical Activity:
1. Warm-up
2. Stretch
3. Workout Card: Day 3 – Workout Phase 2

EXERCISE: DAY 3	BEGINNER	MODERATE	ADVANCED
Cardio	#1 x 19 minutes	#2 x 14 minutes	#3 x 11 minutes
Leg Work #3	2 x 10 times	2 x 15 times	2 x 20 times
Arm Work #5	2 x 10 times	2 x 15 times	2 x 20 times
Ab Work #4 & 5	2 x 10 times	2 x 15 times	2 x 20 times
Ball Work #1 & 4	2 x 10 times	2 x 15 times	2 x 20 times

DAY 4: GENTLENESS AND GOODNESS

Promise: *"But whoso hath this world's good, and seeth his brother have need, and shutteth up his bowels of compassion from him, how dwelleth the love of God in him? My little children let us not love in word, neither in tongue; but in deed and in truth. And hereby we know that we are of the truth, and shall assure our hearts before him. For if our heart condemn us, God is greater than our heart, and knoweth all things"* (1John 3:17-20).

Practice: To sum up the moral excellence of gentleness and the willingness to help others in goodness, this combination would be best described as compassion. As we follow Jesus' ministry, we see that He was moved with compassion on multiple occasions. The moral excellence of His character would not allow Him to ignore those in need just because He was serving them in multiple capacities. Jesus fed the people with the bread of the Word *and* with the bread of the land. He did not abandon them in their time of need simply because He had already spent valuable time and energy teaching and healing them. In Matthew 9:36, when Jesus saw the multitude and they had fainted and were scattered about without guidance, He said to His disciples, *"The harvest truly is plenteous, but the labourers are few; Pray ye therefore the Lord of the harvest, that he will send forth labourers into his harvest."* There are numerous accounts of the King of kings and Lord of lords moving in a spirit of compassion. Jesus met the needs of the people without discrimination or taking a criminal background check. He saw each need and met each need. In faith, they approached Him with many needs, and He acknowledged them. The major missing element in our society is a broad scope of compassion through moral excellence and a willingness to help those in need.

Charity should begin at home. Some people neglect close relatives for many reasons. The needs of these people may or may not be materialistic. Some people need attention while others need companionship. Some people need a word of encouragement or advice, but because of past issues we ignore their cries for help. Sure, we will give a stranger lurking at the gas station a dollar or two, but that is easy when you compare it to spending a few hours with a mentally or emotionally challenged loved one.

The dynamic duo of gentleness and goodness are the seeds of the fruit of the spirit. These seeds are often spewed out. The activation and exercise of this spiritual fruit takes love, longsuffering, and joy and peace if it is to be given in genuine gladness and out of concern for others. Let us take inventory of our lives and the lives of those around us. Today, let us sew some seeds of the spiritual fruits of goodness and gentleness into the lives of wayward teens. Make a phone call or house call to that family member or friend that you have decided is too much work or too far gone. Lend a helping hand to a charitable organization or to your local church, but only after there is no more family work to be done. This includes aunts, uncles, nieces, nephews, parents, grandparents, children, grandchildren, or anyone with whom you share blood, who needs your attention. Give that attention without judgment or fear.

Prayer: Thank you, Lord Jesus, for having compassion on the multitudes and having compassion on me. Fill me, Lord Jesus, with the fruits of gentleness and goodness, that I might live in moral excellence with a willingness to help others, especially my family members. I know that I have struggled in the past with developing the compassion I need to be strong enough to move past selfishness, but you have sent me as a demonstration of how we are to love, to move, and to serve those in need. Forgive me for the times I have failed to extend compassion to a loved one, friend, or stranger.

I pray, as Jesus told His disciplines to pray, that I am sent out as a laborer on behalf of the Lord of the harvest. As I go out, let me not forget your loving-kindness and mercy toward me, so that I may minister well to others. I have received your gifts of love, joy, and peace freely. Let me not forget the torment and pain that consumes a life lived outside of Christ. With this recollection, grant me an urgency to enter into the harvest with the compassion of the Holy Spirit.

Psalm 145:7-10: *"They shall abundantly utter the memory of thy great goodness, and shall sing of thy righteousness. The LORD is gracious, and full of compassion; slow to anger, and of great mercy. The LORD is good to all: and his tender mercies are over all his works. All thy works shall praise thee, O LORD; and thy saints shall bless thee."*

Physical Activity:

1. Warm-up
2. Stretch
3. Workout Card: Day 4 – Workout Phase 2

EXERCISE: DAY 4	BEGINNER	MODERATE	ADVANCED
Cardio #4	2 x 25 non-stop	7 minutes	10 minutes
Leg Work #4	2 x 10 times	2 x 15 times	2 x 20 times
Arm Work #1 & 2	2 x 10 times	2 x 15 times	2 x 20 times
Ab Work #3 & 4	2 x 10 times	2 x 15 times	2 x 20 times
Ball Work #1 & 5	2 x 10 times	2 x 15 times	2 x 20 times

DAY 5: FAITH

Promise: *"Wherefore seeing we also are compassed about with so great a cloud of witnesses, **let us lay aside every weight**, and the sin which doth so easily beset us, and **let us run with patience the race that is set before us, Looking unto Jesus the author and finisher of our faith;** who for the joy that was set before him endured the cross, despising the shame, and is set down at the right hand of the throne of God"* (Hebrews 12:1-2).

Practice: *"Now faith is the substance of things hoped for, the evidence of things not seen"* (Hebrews 11:1). Faith is an action and a reaction. James reminds us that faith without works is dead. As a shepherd boy, David demonstrated that we have to at least show up to the fight and throw the stone. In other words, faith has only whatever limitations *you* put on it. Faith is much larger than what is produced by our hopes. Faith is a daily and consequential walk. Hebrew 11:1 outlines the great faith of those who perfectly executed it. Active faith is not only a belief in a resurrected Christ. It is trusting Christ with your life and His plans for it.

I remember my mother quoting Psalm 20:7 from the time I was five years old: *"Some trust in chariots, and some in horses: but we will remember the name of the LORD our God. They are brought down and fallen: but we are risen, and stand upright. Save, LORD: let the king hear us when we call."* I remember thinking to myself, "Who has a chariot or a horse, and who would trust in a horse and chariot?" I never posed this question to my mother but rather pondered the confusing quote to myself. As I began to grow in my faith, I learned that chariots and horses in that time were of great value. Today, we have chariots and horses called bank accounts, CDs, mutual funds, stock and bonds, property, and jewelry. Now those are true modern-day chariots.

While our faith takes us to church on Sundays, and maybe even Wednesdays, our true trust and expectation typically lies in our titles, paychecks, and circles of friends. However, we must look to and keep our hope and trust in Jesus Christ who is the author and finisher of our faith. We can trust solely in Him because He is seated at the right hand of the Father watching over all of our affairs. Through the power of His Holy Spirit, it is God who blesses our homes and keeps our families together. It is the Holy Spirit who takes our loved ones to and fro in safety. You can rest assured by faith that your prayers move much faster than your vehicle. You can trust that God will keep you and bless you securely in old age with love, laughter, good health, and family. These are never listed in the investment portfolios offered by large securities firms. Consider the plight of those well-vested in Enron and make an investment in the kingdom of God today. The saints of old had retirement accounts with God and, much like my mother, they received daily dividends on Earth and shall continue to receive them throughout eternity. Do you have a retirement account with God? You should try one today! Trust in Him and make a spiritual deposit of faith and trust in Jesus Christ.

Prayer: Lord God Almighty, I thank you for showing us so many examples of the benefits of trusting, believing, and having faith in you. Bless my unbelief and fill me with a great manifestation of the fruit of faith. I know that without faith it is impossible to please you, and I want you to be pleased with all that I do. I ask that you remain in my life from this moment forward. I ask you to stir up a radical Holy Ghost boldness in me so that I can speak to the mountains in my life and watch them move. By faith, Father, I ask you to bless me right now with more trust and faith so that your will is the foundation of my life.

Psalm 118:6-9: *"The LORD is on my side; I will not fear: what can man do unto me? The LORD taketh my part with them that help me: therefore shall I see my desire upon them that hate me. It is better to trust in the LORD than to put confidence in man. It is better to trust in the LORD than to put confidence in princes."*

Physical Activity:
1. Warm-up
2. Stretch
3. Workout Card: Day 5 – Workout Phase 2

EXERCISE: DAY 3	BEGINNER	MODERATE	ADVANCED
Cardio	#1 x 20 minutes	#2 x 15 minutes	#3 x 10 minutes
Leg Work #5	2 x 10 times	2 x 15 times	2 x 20 times
Arm Work #3 & 4	2 x 10 times	2 x 15 times	2 x 20 times
Ab Work #5 & 1	2 x 10 times	2 x 15 times	2 x 20 times
Ball Work #1 & 2	2 x 10 times	2 x 15 times	2 x 20 times

DAY 6: MEEKNESS

Promise: *"Put them in mind to be subject to principalities and powers, to obey magistrates, to be ready to every good work, to speak evil of no man, to be no brawlers, but gentle, shewing all meekness unto all men. For we ourselves also were sometimes foolish, disobedient, deceived, serving divers lusts and pleasures, living in malice and envy, hateful, and hating one another. But after that the kindness and love of God our Saviour toward man appeared, Not by works of righteousness which we have done, but according to his mercy he saved us, by the washing of regeneration, and renewing of the Holy Ghost"* (Titus 3:1-5).

Practice: Without the spirit of meekness, how soon we forget how far we have come and the wonderful transformations Christ has made in our lives. Meekness comes in at number eight as a true indication of the fruit of the spirit. This meekness is qualified through the true humility of remembering the empty, lost, miserable person we were before our encounter with Christ. As we begin to mature, we realize that our actions warranted the death penalty. It was a saving grace that spared us, and not our works of righteousness. False humility is easily revealed through selfish, haughty, and prideful acts. Let us walk in the spirit of meekness, sharing our testimonies of transformation with others. We overcome by the blood of the Lamb and by the word of our testimonies.

Testify of a humbling experience. Declare the marvelous works of the Lord in your life. Share a story of God's deliverance, favor, or breakthrough in your life. Watch what you say and how you judge others. Be gentle and understanding, hoping and expecting a positive outcome for others. Celebrate the

113

victories of others and encourage them in challenges. Anyone, no matter his walk, title, or talk, who confesses the Lord Jesus Christ as his Savior is immediately engaged in a battle over his faith. The last thing we need in the body of Christ is dissention and discord among ourselves. Walk in the spirit of meekness and you will not fulfill the lusts of the flesh. Paul must have been aware of the history of the men he addresses in this letter to Titus. This letter specifically instructs those who were to become elders and bishops. Paul had to step on some toes to remind them of how they were so that, in meekness, they could serve God and His people.

Prayer: Father God, you have been so good to me and you always remember me. In my lowest points, you have sent a word of encouragement through a sermon, phone call, text message, or even email. Help me to reciprocate the encouragement that we need in the body of Christ. Help me to meditate on Titus 3 so that I may be a great ambassador for Christ. Put me in remembrance of the grace, mercy, and compassion that you constantly bestow on me, so that I may also show it to others. Create in me a clean and meek heart and renew a compassionate and loving spirit in me. Lord, send the anointing oil of the Holy Spirit to rest upon me so that I can meet and minister to people wherever they are. Help me to pray fervently and effectively for those who are going through difficult times. Give me a divine strategy developed in Godly wisdom and knowledge to help others make it over spiritual hurdles and stumbling blocks. Lord, I need a fresh anointing every day. Lord, I want to be whole and complete, so fill me with the fruit of compassion. Through seed planting and a watering of your Word, may you bring a full increase to the lives of others. Thank you, Lord. I love you. I need you. Amen.

Psalm 1:1-3: *"Blessed is the man that walketh not in the counsel of the ungodly, nor standeth in the way of sinners, nor sitteth in the seat of the scornful. But his delight is in the law of the LORD; and in his law doth he meditate day and night. And he shall be like a tree planted by the rivers of water, that bringeth forth his fruit in his season; his leaf also shall not wither; and whatsoever he doeth shall prosper."*

Physical Activity:
1. Warm-up
2. Stretch
3. Workout Card: Day 6 – Workout Phase 2

EXERCISE: DAY 6	BEGINNER	MODERATE	ADVANCED
Cardio #4	25 non-stop	7 minutes	10 minutes
Cardio #5	10 minutes	15 minutes	20 minutes
Leg Work #1	2 x 10 times	2 x 15 times	2 x 20 times
Arm Work #5	2 x 10 times	2 x 15 times	2 x 20 times
Ab Work #1 & 2	2 x 10 times	2 x 15 times	2 x 20 times
Ball Work #1 & 3	2 x 10 times	2 x 15 times	2 x 20 times

DAY 7: TEMPERANCE

Promise: *"Whereby are given unto us exceeding great and precious promises: that by these ye might be partakers of the divine nature, having escaped the corruption that is in the world through lust. And beside this, giving all diligence, add to your faith virtue; and to virtue knowledge; And to knowledge temperance; and to temperance patience; and to patience godliness; And to godliness brotherly kindness; and to brotherly kindness charity"* (2 Peter 1:4-7).

Practice: Temperance is the most difficult fruit of the spirit to master. Temperance is self-control, and, because of the complexity of the "individual," it takes years to master oneself. As human beings, we are constantly changing and adjusting to new trends and societal fads. Now add to that humanity the elements of the spirit. One of the greatest types of knowledge one can attain is that of self-knowledge. How do you learn to control yourself when you are constantly changing? While we may master a few things in our lives, the human psyche is a lot of work. All in all, Paul said it best when he described himself as pressing toward the higher calling that he had in Christ Jesus. This indicates that Paul realized that he would never attain the full perfection of Christ, but that he would move toward that perfection day by day. There are so many areas in our lives that are affected by self-control, or the lack of it. Many people struggle with fitness and exercise because of the self-control and discipline it demands. Unlike the discipline needed to earn an education or maintain a career, exercise requires that you inflict what sometimes seems like punishment on your own body. However, exercise, next to fasting, is the best way to bring your flesh under subjection so that it does not rule over you. The spirit is willing but the flesh is weak. You know what is best for you as far as your health.

You know that you should exercise and make healthy food choices, but your body sends these messages to your brain: "I don't feel like it today." "I want some more cake and ice cream." "I don't like water and vegetables, so give me some fried chicken."

The words of primary school children—*feel*, *like*, and *want*—have caused many adults to become mediocre about moving forward in the things of God and the things of life. Wherein the spirit of God is willing to help you, you must put forth the effort. In order to be successful, create a solid plan for your efforts and surround yourself with accountability. This makes a big difference. We have so many plans, ideas, and desires for ourselves locked up in our daily thought processes. If we take these thoughts, write them down, develop a plan, and enlist the help of a partner who is willing to be devoted to our cause, we should begin to see our hopes take shape. We will see the fruit of our efforts. Proverbs 14:23 states that in all labor there is profit, but the talk of the lips leads only to penury, which is poverty, deficit, and lack. Let us exercise self-control in those things that will produce a good harvest in our lives. Let us do those things that we do not like, feel, or want to do, all to the glory of God and for the better execution of self-control in our lives.

Prayer: Father God, I thank you for the completion of another seven days. I thank you for showing me, in detail, your character through your Holy Spirit. I thank you for manifesting the nine fruits of your Holy Spirit in me so that I may be whole, complete, and lacking in nothing. I pray for the fruit of temperance to accomplish the will of your

Holy Spirit through my physical actions. I thank you for more discipline and clarity in studying your Word. I thank you for being more effective and diligent in my prayer life. I thank you for love, joy, peace, the compassion of gentleness and goodness, faith, meekness, and temperance. Lord let me walk, talk, breathe, and move in all of the fruit of the Holy Spirit so that, like Abraham, I can be blessed to be a blessing to many nations, accomplishing your full will for my life. Lord, I thank you for the transformations you have made in my body and in my attitude over the last fourteen days. I am a new creature in Christ. My attitude and reactions have changed and are looking more and more like you, physically and spiritually. I thank you, Lord, for the balance that you have provided to me through praise and worship and the fruits of the spirit. Amen.

Psalm 104:1-5: *"Bless the LORD, O my soul. O LORD my God, thou art very great; thou art clothed with honour and majesty. Who coverest thyself with light as with a garment: who stretchest out the heavens like a curtain: Who layeth the beams of his chambers in the waters: who maketh the clouds his chariot: who walketh upon the wings of the wind: Who maketh his angels spirits; his ministers a flaming fire: Who laid the foundations of the earth, that it should not be removed for ever."*

Physical Activity:

1. Warm-up
2. Stretch
3. Workout Card: Day 7 – Rest!

EXERCISE: DAY 7	BEGINNER	MODERATE	ADVANCED
	REST	REST	REST

Day 7: Remember the Sabbath day and keep it holy, and God will remember you. God rested on the seventh day, and so should you!

Week 3

Fruit of Obedience

The third "peace" of our provisional pineapple is the fruit of obedience. Obedience is a major portion of the Christian life, for through it we find protection, revelation, blessings, favor, and our purpose and destiny. God is constantly communicating His perfect will for our lives through the voice of His Holy Spirit, His word, His prophets, and the things He allows to happen in our lives. Obedience means to submit, comply, heed, to conform, and to listen attentively. In laying out this definition, we see how many could be "called" while only a few are chosen. How can you submit, comply, heed, or conform if you never hear intelligently or listen attentively? There are so many things drowning out God's expressed will for our lives. Our cell phones, satellite radios, television, the internet, meetings, sporting events—all of life's constantly growing and expanding forms of communication constantly block the one and only vital voice of our soul.

Obedience is developed by first learning and discerning what it is that God would have us do. Some of the things we know God requires can be found in the outline of His word or in a sermon preached in church. Most of these things are for our own good, our growth, maturity, and quality of life. However, there is another level of obedience that requires extreme devotion to God, an election of Him over your greatest desire and all you have ever known. The obedience that produced pineapples in the jungle requires silence in a world driven by subliminal messages and blended noise. Allow Jesus to minister the will of the Father for your life. In stillness and quietude, you will hear the voice of the Lord and discern His will for your life. Upon hearing God's voice, you will have the zeal to finally move in obedience with the swiftness of Abraham, knowing that God will provide you with a ram in the bush, pineapples in the jungle, or an even greater boldness for His kingdom. The words "obey God" are a subject and verb that make a complete sentence and a complete command. Does this sentence offend you or move you? The answer to this question will determine your readiness to move forward in obedience.

DAY 1: PROTECTION

Promise: *"When thou passest through the waters, I will be with thee; and through the rivers, they shall not overflow thee: when thou walkest through the fire, thou shalt not be burned; neither shall the flame kindle upon thee. For I am the LORD thy God, the Holy One of Israel, thy Saviour"* (Isaiah 43:2-3).

Practice: Every day we hear of terrorism, global warming, skyrocketing gas prices, corrupt government officials, poor health care, and no retirement funds, just to name a few national challenges. We need to look no further than the local evening news to find the most horrible events only a few doors down in our own neighborhoods. God has promised us that if we believe in the resurrected Christ and put our trust and confidence in Him that He will be with us. Even if the believer feels lost amid the storms of life, we believe and trust in the only risen Savior of the world. There are not even claims of another self-resurrected Savior. So in this confidence, we send our children off to school, we depart to work, leave our homes, and enter into deep waters, winding rivers, and blazing fire each and every day. We rest in the blessed assurance that no matter what a day brings forth, God is with us because we have heard His voice and accepted the perfect sacrifice of His only begotten son, Jesus Christ. When we reject God and His gift, what, then, is our protection? Where, then, is our hope? How anxious a life lived outside of the protection of the blood of Jesus Christ must be.

In the bustle of things, not only can we miss the voice and will of God, but our realities are temporarily quieted, and in this moment we find a false sense of peace. This is what makes reality television and soap operas so popular. They do one of

123

two things for individuals, maybe both. These shows allow people to take their minds off of their own realities or validate some form of normalcy in them.

Today, let us rest assured that there is truth, value, and protection in an obedient relationship with God. Let us remember those who are highly anxious, troubled, and tormented about many things. Let us pray for those individuals today. Let us minister the Word of God to someone who may be weary and tired of being flooded with daily problems or moral compromise. Today, let us share the good news that there is a final resort called Salvation and that it has vacancies for those who labor and are heavily laden. Be someone's travel agent today. Book them a vacation of permanent restoration through the number one carrier of souls, Jesus Christ.

Prayer: **Father God, I thank you for protection in obedience. I pray for much fruit to come forth in my life and in the lives of those around me with every act of obedience. Help me to always remember that you are with me, even until the end of the world. Lord, thank you for maturing me past myself and taking me to another level of fellowship with my fellow man. Give me kind, gentle words of encouragement, filled with wisdom, grace, meekness, and discernment. As I go about my day, I ask that your Holy Spirit go before me and order my steps, and that He minister through me upon my arrival. It is in Jesus' name that I pray for the protection found in obeying your voice and your Word. Bless the name of the Lord! Amen!**

Psalm 91:1-7: *"He that dwelleth in the secret place of the most High shall abide under the shadow of the Almighty. I will say of the LORD, He is my refuge and my fortress: my God; in* *him will I trust. Surely he shall deliver thee from the snare of the fowler, and from the noisome pestilence. He shall cover thee with his feathers, and under his wings shalt thou trust: his truth shall be thy shield and buckler. Thou shalt not be afraid for the terror by night; nor for the arrow that flieth by day; Nor for the pestilence that walketh in darkness; nor for the destruction that wasteth at noonday. A thousand shall fall at thy side, and ten thousand at thy right hand; but it shall not come nigh thee."*

Physical Activity:
1. Warm-up
2. Stretch
3. Workout Card: Day 1 – Workout Phase 3

EXERCISE: DAY 1	BEGINNER	MODERATE	ADVANCED
Cardio	#1 x 15 minutes	#2 x 10 minutes	#3 x 7 minutes
Leg Work #1	3 x 10 times	3 x 15 times	3 x 20 times
Arm Work #1 & 2	3 x 10 times	3 x 15 times	3 x 20 times
Ab Work #1 & 2	3 x 10 times	3 x 15 times	3 x 20 times
Ball Work #1 & 2	3 x 10 times	3 x 15 times	3 x 20 times

DAY 2: BETTER THAN SACRIFICE

Promise: *"And Samuel said, Hath the LORD as great delight in burnt offerings and sacrifices, as in obeying the voice of the LORD? Behold, to obey is better than sacrifice, and to hearken than the fat of rams. For rebellion is as the sin of witchcraft, and stubbornness is as iniquity and idolatry. Because thou hast rejected the word of the LORD, he hath also rejected thee from being king"* (1 Samuel 15:22-23).

Practice: If you have children or a pet, or people you are in charge of, you also have rules and expectations that are set in place for an overall benefit. Children are told not to use the stove or to run into the street, and they are expected not to take the car key and start the car, no matter how ready they think they are. Your pet is given borders, perimeters, and limits and is expected to treat its dwelling place like a home, not a backyard. Those whom you may supervise are expected to follow the policies and procedures outlined in the employee handbook and adjust to newly implemented requirements and changes. If all is well and your rules are followed, then this section is not for you and you may move on to day three, but do not skip the exercise.

So, your child uses the stove and the house burns down. You lose everything, you have to stay with family members and figure out what to do next while the insurance company accuses you of plotting to burn down your own house. Go figure? What excuse would be acceptable for this blatant disobedience?

You have had your family pet for several years and when you return home one day, you discover that it has deliberately destroyed clothing, fine china, and furniture. What rationale would you want to hear?

Your best client just released its contract with your company because specific instructions were not followed in processing its service. What explanation would you accept?

This is how it is when God gives us specific instructions. How many times have you felt the spirit of God moving you to do something over and over again and you did not move? How many times has He told you to apologize for your behavior toward someone and you have refused? Who is it whom He has assigned you to walk with, minister to and serve, but because you did not like His choice, you ignored the assignment? God's foolishness is wiser than we are and His weakness is stronger than we are. You can trust God in even what seems to be foolishness, because you never know what blessing your obedience will bring or the hazard it is allowing you to avoid. Using Samuel, God compares rebellion to witchcraft, and says that stubbornness is as bad as iniquity and idolatry. Today, let us listen, learn, and obey. God is not as interested in many gifts, much praying and fasting, studying and church service. He seeks obedience. Let him find an obedient and willing heart in you today so that your offerings, requests, petitions, and sacrifices may be accepted and not rejected.

Prayer: Father God, if I have been operating in any form of rebellion to your Word, your will for my life, your Holy Spirit, or to any of those you have placed over me, I ask your forgiveness. I repent for being stubborn and resistant to your commands for my life. Father, I pray that you will help me to be better prepared to move in your will this time. Lord, I ask you to make me spiritually sensitive to any form of rebellion or stubbornness that may creep into my mind or actions. Allow me to take authority over these things and execute obedience. Father, I pray for more boldness and courage to move in obedience, even when it seems foolish. Lord, fix every situation that has gone out of order because of my disobedience. I am asking you for another chance to obey your voice and keep your commands, for in them is more abundant life. Thank you, Father, for hearing me, showing me my errors, and allowing me to correct them. Thank you for your patience with me. Help me show mercy to others as you have shown mercy to me. Amen.

Psalm 103:8-13: *"The LORD is merciful and gracious, slow to anger, and plenteous in mercy. He will not always chide: neither will he keep his anger for ever. He hath not dealt with us after our sins; nor rewarded us according to our iniquities. For as the heaven is high above the earth, so great is his mercy toward them that fear him. As far as the east is from the west, so far hath he removed our transgressions from us. Like as a father pitieth his children, so the LORD pitieth them that fear him."*

Physical Activity:

1. Warm-up
2. Stretch
3. Workout Card: Day 2 – Workout Phase 3

EXERCISE: DAY 2	BEGINNER	MODERATE	ADVANCED
Cardio #5	13 minutes	18 minutes	23 minutes
Leg Work #2	3 x 10 times	3 x 15 times	3 x 20 times
Arm Work #3 & 4	3 x 10 times	3 x 15 times	3 x 20 times
Ab Work #2 & 3	3 x 10 times	3 x 15 times	3 x 20 times
Ball Work #1 & 3	3 x 10 times	3 x 15 times	3 x 20 times

DAY 3: ANSWERED PRAYERS

Promise: *"If my people, which are called by my name, shall humble themselves, and pray, and seek my face, and turn from their wicked ways; then will I hear from heaven, and will forgive their sin, and will heal their land"* (2 Chronicles 7:14).

Practice: God is a prayer-answering God. However, many prayers go unanswered because of disobedience. The book of James outlines the prayers that bring forth much fruit: *"Confess your faults one to another, and pray one for another, that ye may be healed. The effectual fervent prayer of a righteous man availeth much" (James 5:16).* This means that prayer should be concise and specific, as well as continual. These concise, specific, continual prayers must be made by the righteous. A lack of any of the aforementioned adjectives could easily render a prayer-life stagnant and unfruitful. Likewise, it is with our promise for today.

God's own chosen people are described here as "needing" to humble themselves, pray, seek God's face, and turn from their wicked ways so that the land might be healed. Our land is not sick because of the unrighteous and the sinner, it is sick because of those who are "called" by God's name and are rebellious, wicked, and disobedient. God is informing His people of what it will take to make Him hear from Heaven. This prerequisite has not changed over the centuries. We still need to obey, seek His face, humble ourselves, turn from wickedness, and pray humbly before God. God wants to forgive our sins and heal our land, but we will not forgive each other.

Unforgiveness is another prayer blocker. Attempting to pray while harboring unforgiveness in your heart is like trying to speak to your spouse through a six-inch concrete wall. God finds favor in the simplicity of righteous living. Please do not confuse righteous living with perfection. These are different things. Righteous living means making a conscientious effort to do what is right while attempting to correct any wrong. When we approach God the right way in prayer, His response is much like the response of the father of an obedient, respectful, straight-A student who is the captain of the football team when he asks for five dollars. God will not withhold any good thing from those whom He loves.

Today, let us approach God's throne in right living. Let's check every aspect of our lives and do away with habits, activities, and people who interfere with right living. Let us get our houses in order so that, when we pray, God is anxious to answer us.

Prayer: Lord God, I thank you that I am yours. I thank you that through your love, you have sent your Word to inform me of what it takes for you to hear me and heal the land. Father God, on this day I give the Holy Spirit complete control of my life. I put aside all that comes between you and me when I pray. Give me the wisdom, knowledge, and understanding that I need to be effectual and fervent in my prayer-life. I continue to pray and ask for an even bolder sense of obedience so that I may do your will. Lord, grant me a praying, obedient spirit so that your will shall be glorified and magnified through answered prayer.

Psalm 145: 18-19: *"The LORD is nigh unto all them that call upon him, to all that call upon him in truth. He will fulfill the desire of them that fear him: he also will hear their cry, and will save them."*

Physical Activity:
1. Warm-up
2. Stretch
3. Workout Card: Day 3 – Workout Phase 3

EXERCISE: DAY 3	BEGINNER	MODERATE	ADVANCED
Cardio	#1 x 16 minutes	#2 x 11 minutes	#3 x 8 minutes
Leg Work #3	3 x 10 times	3 x 15 times	3 x 20 times
Arm Work #5	3 x 10 times	3 x 15 times	3 x 20 times
Ab Work #4 & 5	3 x 10 times	3 x 15 times	3 x 20 times
Ball Work #1 & 4	3 x 10 times	3 x 15 times	3 x 20 times

DAY 4: ELEVATION

Promise: *"And it shall come to pass, if thou shalt hearken diligently unto the voice of the LORD thy God, to observe and to do all his commandments which I command thee this day, that the LORD thy God will set thee on high above all nations of the earth"* (Deuteronomy 28:1).

Practice: If you obey the Lord, He will set you in high places and blow your mind with His awesome wonder. Joseph, though thrown into slavery by his brothers and unfamiliar with the laws of the land, is familiar with the sin of adultery and eludes Potiphar's wife's advances in fear of God and in obedience to Him. After fasting for forty days and forty nights, Jesus stands on God's Word through obedience, though satan attempts to make Him fall. David, when given the opportunity to kill his archenemy Saul, was obedient and controlled his sword.

The obedience of these men not only spared them from destructive, self-gratifying decisions, it also took them to places of elevation. Joseph, though thrown into prison, was later vindicated and named second only to Pharaoh in power over Egypt. Jesus was immediately attended to by an angel. He was crucified, but now He is the King of Glory. David went on to become the king of Israel and was called a man after God's own heart. Your obedience to God's Word can take you to places of elevation and promotion. Promotion comes from the Lord. He puts one up and takes another down. If you are looking to be promoted in some aspect of your life, remember the process from hardship to great heights can be painful and difficult. But be of good cheer because when you go through obeying God, you can expect eventual elevation.

Prayer: Lord, I thank you for where I am and how far you have brought me. I do not take this process of growth and development lightly. Help me, Lord, to face my challenges in obedience to you without wavering toward the convenient but detrimental choice of the moment. Teach me, oh Lord, to make decisions based on eternity and not for reasons that are convenient to me. I know, Lord, that there are great things in store for me because you are faithful and just, tried and true. No one can love me or bless me like you. While you are working your perfect work of elevating me, fill me with gentleness, goodness, meekness, and humility. Amen.

Psalm 18:30-34: *"As for God, his way is perfect: the word of the LORD is tried: he is a buckler to all those that trust in him. For who is God save the LORD? or who is a rock save our God? It is God that girdeth me with strength, and maketh my way perfect. He maketh my feet like hinds' feet, and setteth me upon my high places. He teacheth my hands to war, so that a bow of steel is broken by mine arms."*

Physical Activity:
1. Warm-up
2. Stretch
3. Workout Card: Day 4 – Workout Phase 3

EXERCISE: DAY 4	BEGINNER	MODERATE	ADVANCED
Cardio #4	3 x 25 non-stop	7 minutes	10 minutes
Leg Work #4	3 x 10 times	3 x 15 times	3 x 20 times
Arm Work #1 & 2	3 x 10 times	3 x 15 times	3 x 20 times
Ab Work #3 & 4	3 x 10 times	3 x 15 times	3 x 20 times
Ball Work #1 & 5	3 x 10 times	3 x 15 times	3 x 20 times

DAY 5: HEALING

Promise: *"Elisha sent a messenger to him, saying, "Go and wash in the Jordan seven times, and your flesh will be restored to you and you will be clean." But Naaman was furious and went away and said, "Behold, I thought, 'He will surely come out to me and stand and call on the name of the LORD his God, and wave his hand over the place and cure the leper'"* (2 Kings 5:10-11, NASB).

Practice: Healing of all sorts may be found in obedience to God's Word. This includes physical healing in your body. In the above text, Naaman was seeking healing from one of the most deadly diseases of that time. Naaman, however, already had made up in his mind exactly how his healing should take place. The demand for his idea of healing almost caused Naaman to miss his healing altogether. Thank God that he had wise counsel to encourage him to obey.

Good health can be found in obedience and self-control. The fact is that our health is directly related to our food choice and level of activity, and we must remember this. We often pass over the fruit of the land for the fat of fast food. Some people may not consider making poor food choices disobedient. However, when you know better and choose not to do better, that is equal to disobedience. God has shown you how to be healthy and healed, but it is up to you to take action. You cannot be picky and choosy about how your healing will take place. By faith, we trust that God sends healing and deliverance, not hurt or harm. We can trust that even when God's solutions to our illnesses look murky and dirty, there is restoration on the other side because of our obedience. It is through rebellion that we miss the mark and remain in a state of sickness.

Let's meditate on the healing power of obedience today. Let Jehovah Rapha, our healer, come in and do a thorough spiritual and physical examination. Whatever the Lord says to do, you can trust that He will make a way and make you white as snow.

Prayer: Oh Lord God, you are my healer and my helper. I embrace the wisdom, knowledge, and understanding you have given to me and with which you have surrounded me. Help me to use the information I am given to take better care of myself and be a better steward over my health. I pray for temperance, self-control of the Holy Spirit, for without it I can do very little on my own. Lord, I want to prosper and be in good health as my soul begins to prosper. Preserve my life, oh Lord, from untimely death and poor health. As I rapidly complete this twenty-eight days of fitness, I pray that this is just the beginning of a new lifestyle for me. Thank you, Lord, for a new lease on life and a new opportunity to be a better, whole, and complete Christian. Hallelujah for Heaven-based health!

Psalm 103:1-5: *"Bless the LORD, O my soul: and all that is within me, bless his holy name. Bless the LORD, O my soul, and forget not all his benefits: Who forgiveth all thine iniquities; who healeth all thy diseases; Who redeemeth thy life from destruction; who crowneth thee with lovingkindness and tender mercies; Who satisfieth thy mouth with good things; so that thy youth is renewed like the eagle's."*

Physical Activity:
1. Warm-up
2. Stretch
3. Workout Card: Day 5 – Workout Phase 3

EXERCISE: DAY 5	BEGINNER	MODERATE	ADVANCED
Cardio	#1 x 23 minutes	#2 x 18 minutes	#3 x 11 minutes
Leg Work #5	3 x 10 times	3 x 15 times	3 x 20 times
Arm Work #3 & 4	3 x 10 times	3 x 15 times	3 x 20 times
Ab Work #5 & 1	3 x 10 times	3 x 15 times	3 x 20 times
Ball Work #1 & 2	3 x 10 times	3 x 15 times	3 x 20 times

DAY 6: VICTORY

Promise: *"The LORD shall cause thine enemies that rise up against thee to be smitten before thy face: they shall come out against thee one way, and flee before thee seven ways"* (Deuteronomy 28:7).

Practice: There is great victory in obedience to God's Word, and our enemies are almost always destroyed. Haman, in the book of Esther, claims that all of the favor the king bestowed upon him meant nothing so long as the Jew Mordecai sat at the king's gate. Haman's wife and friends persuaded him to build gallows fifty feet high to hang the innocent Mordecai upon. Mordecai must have possessed great authority and power. Not only was Haman utterly disgusted at the mere sight of him, he plotted to hang the man and wipe out an entire people.

Queen Ester was secure and well-favored by the king. Queen Ester, Mordecai's niece, matriculated to the throne by pleasing the king and obeying her uncle's orders not to disclose her Jewish heritage. Ester obeyed the voice of her uncle once more when he brought to her attention Haman's plan to destroy him and the Jewish people. Ester called a three-day fast and put her life on the line to gain the favor and mercy of the king regarding the decree of destruction upon her uncle and her people. Without saying a word, God favored Ester through the king of the land and Haman was hung on the same gallows he erected for Mordecai. The word *God* is not mentioned in the book of Ester, nor is there any reference to God. However, we see God move through the characters in this story. Ester's obedience and loyalty was to her uncle, and this gave an entire people victory in what seemed like a hopeless situation.

Seven is the number of completion. In the above Scriptural promise, I believe the seven-way fleeing depicts a complete destruction of our enemies when we obey God through good counselors. In the multitude of counselors, there is safety. Do you despise or embrace good counsel? Have you become weary of the counsel of your elderly parents or other family members? Think again and humble yourself, because these people are full of experience, if not wisdom and counsel. They can tell you how to make your enemies flee before you seven ways. Let us seek out the counsel and conversation of those who are older and wiser and know the Lord.

Prayer: Thank you, Lord, for victory over my enemies and having seven ways of dealing with them. I will not be afraid to obey Godly counsel in the heat of the battle, for I now realize that you can and will speak to me through others. I embrace the elders of my family, and I will not reject them in their old age. I pray patience, compassion, and understanding to deposit love and attention while drawing on age-old wisdom and counsel. I thank you for my elders, for they know the story of who I am because of who they are in you. I pray for the health of my elders and a high quality of life for them, even in old age. When they retire back to you, it is I who will take their place in the hope that I can continue to share the story of Christ in us, the hope of Glory. Amen.

Psalm 71:17 *"O God, thou hast taught me from my youth: and hitherto have I declared thy wondrous works. Now also when I am old and greyheaded, O God, forsake me not; until I have shewed thy strength unto this generation, and thy power to every one that is to come."*

Physical Activity:

1. Warm-up
2. Stretch
3. Workout Card: Day 6 – Workout Phase 3

EXERCISE: DAY 6	BEGINNER	MODERATE	ADVANCED
Cardio #4	25 non-stop	7 minutes	10 minutes
Cardio #5	10 minutes	15 minutes	20 minutes
Leg Work #1	3 x 10 times	3 x 15 times	3 x 20 times
Arm Work #5	3 x 10 times	3 x 15 times	3 x 20 times
Ab Work #1 & 2	3 x 10 times	3 x 15 times	3 x 20 times
Ball Work #1 & 3	3 x 10 times	3 x 15 times	3 x 20 times

DAY 7: MAJOR BREAKTHROUGH PROVISION

Promise: *"Then Elijah said to her, "Do not fear; go, do as you have said, but make me a little bread cake from it first and bring it out to me, and afterward you may make one for yourself and for your son"* (1 Kings 17:13).

Practice: This is another admirable act of obedience shown in a story that took place in the middle of a famine. The widow informed Elijah of her intentions of making a final cake of bread for her and her son to eat before she succumbed to death due to the famine. Elijah, a complete stranger, yet a man of God, then turns to her and says to trust him and to feed him first and that there would be enough for the two of them. The widow moves in obedience, and her household is fed for many days. How many of you would have died from starvation after proceeding with your plans of making the bread cake for you and your son? I am thinking that perhaps that would be me. My son is near and dear to my heart. The thought of him starving and then my issuing out first rations of the last of our food to a stranger makes no sense to me. The impracticality of God does not always make sense. Since we have already learned that his foolishness is wiser than we are, we should be ready to move when we are called to do what seems foolish. There is an old pastoral saying: "What does not meet your need, must be your seed." How many times have we consumed the seed of our harvests for lack of faith and trust to sow it back into fertile soil?

Some years ago, long before I was a "Survivor" contestant, I was invited to the church of a widow to be the guest speaker for a conference. I knew this lady well and had made no compensation agreement. After the engagement, she quietly approached me with a jar of quarters, showing me her gratitude for my time and for blessing the people. I looked into her eyes, and, with humble respect, I rejected the offer of the quarters and told her I would be billing God because I had been on assignment for Him. With much relief, she spoke a blessing over my life and we parted ways. While I was in-flight, I checked my voicemail and heard a message from a media company requesting that my talent be used to shoot several commercials. The job would be the following week and the payout for the shoot was over $1,000. I am sure that there must have been only about $50 worth of quarters in the jar the widow had to give. But, because I waited on the hand of His provision, I was given twenty times more. I sowed a portion of the proceeds of the commercial back into the widow's house.

Today, let us be sensitive to those whom we serve. Let us look for opportunities to use God's charge card account. He has no limits or account maximums. When we cannot afford it, we can put it on His account, and, when the bill is paid, we will find a larger and more rewarding amount.

Prayer: Lord God Almighty, you are worthy to be praised! You have brought me through twenty-one days so far. I love you, and I thank you for teaching me all of your marvelous ways. I am three times complete and now ready for the final phase in this 28-day plan. Thank you for the provisions you make for me each day and night. Help me to be faithful and always live right. I am looking at my body, and it is getting trim. I had long given up on ever being thin. I now have a prescription to follow day by day, and it has helped me be successful in many ways. So, I thank you for my prayer time. I thank you for my praise time. I thank you for completing a new me just in time. I thank you for sending me sweet

pineapples in the jungle. Hallelujah! Oh Glory! Hallelujah!
Amen!

Psalm 132: 14-16: *"This is my rest for ever: here will I dwell;
for I have desired it. I will abundantly bless her provision: I will
satisfy her poor with bread. I will also clothe her priests with
salvation: and her saints shall shout aloud for joy."*

Physical Activity:
1. Warm-up
2. Stretch
3. Workout Card: Day 7 – Workout Phase 3

EXERCISE: DAY 7	BEGINNER	MODERATE	ADVANCED
	REST	REST	REST

Day 7—Remember the Sabbath day and to keep it holy,
and God will remember you. God rested on the seventh day,
and so should you!

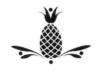

Week 4

Fruit of Sacrifice

DAY 1: GIVING

Promise: *"If a brother or sister be naked, and destitute of daily food, And one of you say unto them, Depart in peace, be ye warmed and filled; notwithstanding ye give them not those things which are needful to the body; what doth it profit?"* (James 2:15-16).

Practice: With the exception of extraordinarily selfish individuals, it is a natural human reaction to share what we have with others. Sharing brings about an overwhelming sense of joy, bonding, and trust to both the giver and the receiver. In grade school, our teachers would often say when we would attempt to eat candy or snacks in school, "Do you have enough for everyone?" Our classmates would look intensely at the culprit, hoping for a response that would favor the whole class. Rarely did anyone have enough for everyone. The teacher's point to input empathy into the heart of the person indulging in a mid-afternoon snack was duly noted. This line of questioning allowed the person snacking and those watching in hunger to realize how much happier it would be for everyone to participate. We later prided ourselves on being the one who put the smiles on the faces of others by bringing enough to share.

It is so easy to share when you have plenty. You usually never miss it, and it rarely requires much sacrifice on your behalf. The fruit of sacrifice in giving is only produced when you give out of your own need and in a way that might be inconvenient for you.

This was the case with a miracle performed by Jesus in John 6:9. There was a boy who only had five barley loaves and two small fishes. Let's stop there. What would you have done if there were five thousand hungry people and you had a personal pan pizza? Honestly, would you trust the Lord to feed everyone with your small portion? This child had lots of faith, plenty of courage, and, most importantly, he was willing to make a big sacrifice for the crowd. He put his only provision on the line. Jesus expresses concern for those who follow Him and are hungry. He takes personal responsibility for feeing those who follow Him. However, it does take the sacrificial gifts of those within the group to make the Christian experience beneficial for all members. Jesus took the lad's sacrifice of his only food, then blessed and fed everyone present. As a matter of fact, they had plenty left over. The lad was able to eat and got a great return on his investment.

Let us give today, cheerfully, not just what is of convenience, but let us go out of our way to bring about a benefit to all of those around us. Make a sacrifice today that blesses everyone around you. *"But this I say, He which soweth sparingly shall reap also sparingly; and he which soweth bountifully shall reap also bountifully. Every man according as he purposeth in his heart, so let him give; not grudgingly, or of necessity: for God loveth a cheerful giver. And God is able to make all grace abound toward you; that ye, always having all sufficiency in all things, may abound to every good work"* (2 Corinthians 9:6-8).

Prayer: Dear Lord, I thank you for the resources that you have given me. I thank you that, like Abraham, I am blessed to be a blessing to others. Lord, help me to always remember that you bless me so that I may bless others, and we all can bless you for your goodness and mercy. You are Jehovah Jireh, my provider. Help me to remember that I can never lose while giving in the name of Jesus.

Jesus told His disciples that there are many mansions in your house and that he has gone to prepare a place for all of us. Lord, the Earth is yours, and all that I have is on loan from you. I will not forget that from the dust I have come and to dust I will return, taking nothing with me, not even a strip of the physical body I have been given. I pray for the discipline to wear this world like a loose garment so that if I have things I desire, I will be grateful, and, if I never attain certain things, I will still be grateful.

I pray for faith and obedience to give unto you when being led by the Holy Spirit and assisting another in need. Help me, oh Lord, to be content in whatever state I find myself, not aiming for mediocrity, but accepting the fate sometimes associated with righteousness. I trust you, Lord. I trust that all that I have belongs to you. I trust that sacrificial giving in the name of Jesus Christ with love and humility will produce a great harvest for me and all of those around me. Make me a trustworthy servant, oh Lord, and make me faithful over everything you have and will ever trust me

145

with. This is my earnest prayer in the matchless name of Jesus Christ. Amen.

Psalm 37:16: *"A little that a righteous man hath is better than the riches of many wicked."*

Physical Activity:
1. Warm-up
2. Stretch
3. Workout Card: Day 1 – Workout Phase 4

EXERCISE: DAY 1	BEGINNER	MODERATE	ADVANCED
Cardio	#1 x 15 minutes	#2 x 10 minutes	#3 x 7 minutes
Leg Work #1	4 x 10 times	4 x 15 times	4 x 20 times
Arm Work #1 & 2	4 x 10 times	4 x 15 times	4 x 20 times
Ab Work #1 & 2	4 x 10 times	4 x 15 times	4 x 20 times
Ball Work #1 & 2	4 x 10 times	4 x 15 times	4 x 20 times

DAY 2: HELPING

Promise: *"And Jesus answering said, A certain man went down from Jerusalem to Jericho, and fell among thieves, which stripped him of his raiment, and wounded him, and departed, leaving him half dead. And by chance there came down a certain priest that way: and when he saw him, he passed by on the other side. And likewise a Levite, when he was at the place, came and looked on him, and passed by on the other side. But a certain Samaritan, as he journeyed, came where he was: and when he saw him, he had compassion on him, And went to him, and bound up his wounds, pouring in oil and wine, and set him on his own beast, and brought him to an inn, and took care of him. And on the morrow when he departed, he took out two pence, and gave them to the host, and said unto him, Take care of him; and whatsoever thou spendest more, when I come again, I will repay thee. Which now of these three, thinkest thou, was neighbour unto him that fell among the thieves?"* (Luke 10:30-36).

Practice: In the above passage, Jesus describes three different people who could have helped someone in great distress. He describes a church leader who actually avoids the fallen man by crossing to the other side of the street. Another person saw the fallen stranger. He was a Levite. The name translates to "devoted to the Lord." Levites are those who are given, or have given themselves, to the service of the Lord. This Levite was so bold as to get close enough to the fallen man to glimpse the severity of his dilemma, only to walk away, ignoring the stranger's plight by also crossing to the other side of the road. Finally, there is the full description of the true motives and heart of the third passerby, a Samaritan. The noble Samaritan went to the stranger, looked at the situation with compassion and mercy, and proceeded to comfort the "fallen fellowman" without question. He cleaned and dressed his wounds and put him on his own animal to ride. He did not stop there, but, with zeal and passion, took the man to the nearest shelter, paid for his stay and care, and left his credit card for future purchases. The text does not indicate that the fallen man ever asked for help. Jesus ends the parable asking which of these three were more neighborly.

Let us evaluate our own level of helping. The extension of most of our helping ends with priorities and "requests," outlined by our local churches or civic organizations. Helping through the local church and being dependable for your friends, family, and neighbors is noble in and of itself, to say the least. However, let us go beyond giving the sentimental and emotional help that is so easy to express to friends and family. In order to fully enjoy the harvest of the sacrifice of helping, we must contribute at a level that challenges personal convenience and time.

We have the number 911 to offer assistance for those who are really in distress, like the fallen fellow in our parable. While 911 has gotten a bad rap for slow response time and low efficiency, I am very appreciative to live in a society that offers the option of instant human help. I would like to take this moment to acknowledge all of our emergency response personnel for all of your help each and every day. Thank you!

How many rides have you offered to those walking the street? And, I am almost sure that you have never used your credit or debit card to help a complete stranger in need. We all know that there are dangers in picking strangers up off of the street and even in helping others, but what about an elderly person somewhere in your proximity who needs not only the ride, attention, and assistance, but the energy of your youth and vibrancy?

I could go on and on about various ways to offer sacrificial help that often requires more of you than your money. Today's challenge is to move beyond the "easy" help we offer when a request is made, and to move into observational help that could literally change someone's life. Look around, take inventory and take action. By offering multiple forms of sacrificial help, we activate a ripple effect of empathetic intervention that is a healing balm for an injured society while creating a cycle of restitution bound to come back to us or those closest to us. Take a look at the lives of those close to you and look for ways to lighten their heavy loads through being the unsolicited helping hand of Christ.

Prayer: **Father God, we thank you for putting us in a position to really help each other. Help us even now, Lord, to use this gifting to bind our hearts in Christian love and fellowship. In helping others, Father God, help us to spare no expense, giving until the need is met and despair dispelled. Help us to remember that we are blessed with good health and vital resources not to horde or compete with others, but to be a blessing to those in need. Give us wisdom and guidance so that we will know how and when to set borders so that we might never waste our valuable time on manipulators and deceivers.**

Father God, help us not to look for men to appreciate and acknowledge our hard work and efforts, but let us be like David, lifting our eyes to the hills, knowing that our help (and appreciation) comes from you. Help us to do all that we do to your glory and honor and in the name of Jesus Christ. Replenish us so that we will not be weary in well-doing and we will reap a great harvest if we faint not. Remind us daily,

oh Lord, to love our neighbors as we love ourselves. Remind us that the seeds of mercy and grace that we sow will come to harvest in our lives, the lives of our children and loved ones, or even the third and fourth generation. Your Word, oh Lord, is settled in Heaven forever, and your Word says that we will reap what we sow. We pray for the strength, love, compassion, empathy, and resources to sow bountifully in the name of Jesus Christ. Amen.

Psalm 70:1: *"Make haste, O God, to deliver me; make haste to help me, O Lord."*

Physical Activity:
1. Warm-up
2. Stretch
3. Workout Card: Day 2 – Workout Phase 4

EXERCISE: DAY 2	BEGINNER	MODERATE	ADVANCED
Cardio #5	15 minutes	20 minutes	25 minutes
Leg Work #2	4 x 10 times	4 x 15 times	4 x 20 times
Arm Work #3 & 4	4 x 10 times	4 x 15 times	4 x 20 times
Ab Work #2 & 3	4 x 10 times	4 x 15 times	4 x 20 times
Ball Work #1 & 3	4 x 10 times	4 x 15 times	4 x 20 times

DAY 3: TRIBULATION

Promise: *"Then Job arose, and rent his mantle, and shaved his head, and fell down upon the ground, and worshipped, And said, Naked came I out of my mother's womb, and naked shall I return thither: the LORD gave, and the LORD hath taken away; blessed be the name of the LORD. In all this Job sinned not, nor charged God foolishly"* (Job 1:20-22).

Practice: If you are a mature Christian who has been in the faith long enough, then I am sure that there has been a time or two in your walk that you can identify with Job's seemingly needless tribulations. Earlier in the chapter, it is clear that Job is righteous, and he took sacrifice so seriously that he made it a form of preventive insurance. The text indicates that Job would arise early and pray and make sacrifices unto the Lord "just in case" his sons or daughters sinned against God in their hearts. (See Job 1:5). Oftentimes, because we begin our faith in God through loving-kindness, nurturing, and supernatural provision, we are baffled when what appear to be unprovoked pain, trials, and tribulation arise. We follow the Word, we help others, we are faithful to our spouses, diligent in rearing our children, and we still find ourselves looking down the pipeline of disappointment and despair. These trials and challenges can become so harsh and bitter that we want to back out and away from the very faith we once practiced and preached with radical boldness.

If you are new to the faith, this may serve as a reality check: God is not "Santa Claus," nor is He in competition with the world. Only His blessings make us rich and add no sorrow. Though you may experience temporary inconvenience and

151

struggles, these will not hold a permanent position in your life. Therefore, you should not base your walk of faith on anything other than the promises of God. *"These things I have spoken unto you, that in me ye might have peace. In the world ye shall have tribulation: but be of good cheer; I have overcome the world"* (John 16:33). Here, in John, tribulation is confirmed as a part of the Christian walk.

Although it is not fully expressed in the text, Job's irrational faith and confidence in God had to have come about through a lifetime of the demonstrated faithfulness of God toward Job. Job's plight is absolutely shattering. He lost his entire family, with the exception of a lukewarm wife. He lost his power and position. Then, Job's body was struck by satan to the point that his very flesh began to pull away from his bones. Have you ever experienced this level of tribulation, or does it just seem like it? Have you considered God's servant, Job? Have you compared your level of suffering in the faith to that of Job or Jesus? As satan plots around the throne of God, challenging the faithfulness of those who say they love God, he reminds God that the hedge around Job's life and all he owns is so solid that he could never touch him without permission. See Job 1:10. God lowers the hedge and allows this request with limitations on the taking of Job's life and full knowledge of the depth of Job's faithfulness.

In Chapter 9, Job says he wishes that he had an arbitrator, someone, anyone who could plead his flawless righteousness before the living God, but there is no Christ at the right hand of the Father in Job's season of tribulation. The evil one is still up to trying the faithfulness of those fully devoted to the faith as Jesus informs Simon Peter of satan's request and demand for his very life. Even in Jesus' foreknowledge of satan's plots prior to His transfiguration, he intervened through prayer for Simon Peter that his faith might be strong. (See Luke 22:31.)

Jesus is our arbitrator in these days of tribulation. He sits at the right hand of the Father, ensuring that those who confess His Holy name, and who acknowledge redemption by His blood and the power of His resurrection will not face "unnecessary" tribulation. All of the tribulation that we face is to strengthen us, our faith, and even those around us.

We overcome by the word of our testimonies and the blood of the Lamb. There is no *testimony* without a *test*. While tribulation in our lives matures us in many ways, the most important point of it is to stretch, strengthen, and lengthen our faith. For while it appears that through the confusion, heartache, pain, disaster, death, and many other detriments, the warfare is about things and people, it is not. These are mere distractions designed to destroy, dampen, or even weaken your faith. Let us grow in tribulation today. Let us embrace those things that cause us to pray more and reach deeper.

Today, look at your trials and tribulations as elevations and new stages. Grow in your tribulation. Never give up. It is only a test for you to pass and move forward to higher heights and deeper depths. God loves you so much that he is still preparing you for the next level. Press on toward your higher calling, and, if you find yourself living without tribulation, this means perhaps that you may have reached the peak of your calling. Whatever positions you find yourself in, remember that God loves you and that He cares for you. His Word indicates that those whom he loves, He chastens and matures. Search your heart to determine what might shake the foundation of your faith. Begin praying for God to give you serenity and peace no matter what tribulation you are faced with, that you might remain faithful to Him no matter what happens.

Prayer: Father God, thank you for the sobering reality that living the true Christian life often means enduring what seem like unbearable challenges. Give me strength and wisdom, even now, to recognize and appreciate trials and tribulations governed by your guidance and grace. Help me to remember those real life biblical trailblazers who embraced prison, fiery furnaces, lions' dens, flogging, stoning, and even death. Teach me to be bold and confident in my faith no matter what happens to me. I thank you that there is great promise at the end of every trial and time of suffering (1 Peter 5:10).

I trust you Lord. No matter what I face today, let me remember that there are huge rewards for the sacrifice of tribulation. Help me to remember that Job was restored—and given "double for his trouble"; and that Christ rose with all power in His hand, taking full ownership of the realms of death and hell while seated in a position of praise, power, and prominence at the right hand of the Father. Grant me patience in my tribulation and bless any unbelief that may arise. Search my heart and the secret places of my soul, oh God, and shape me and make me into all that you created me to be. Even if it causes me discomfort and pain, Father, I really want to move toward a higher calling. Praise be to God for the growth of my Christian faith through the sacrifice of trials and tribulation. Amen.

Psalm 34:1-8 *"I will bless the LORD at all times: his praise shall continually be in my mouth. My soul shall make her boast in the LORD: the humble shall hear thereof, and be glad. O magnify the LORD with me, and let us exalt his name together. I sought the LORD, and he heard me, and delivered me from all my fears. They looked unto him, and were lightened: and*

*their faces were not ashamed. This poor man cried, and the
LORD heard him, and saved him out of all his troubles. The
angel of the LORD encampeth round about them that fear him,
and delivereth them. O taste and see that the LORD is good:
blessed is the man that trusteth in him."*

Physical Activity:
1. Warm-up
2. Stretch
3. Workout Card: Day 3 – Workout Phase 4

EXERCISE: DAY 3	BEGINNER	MODERATE	ADVANCED
Cardio	#1 x 16 minutes	#2 x 11 minutes	#3 x 8 minutes
Leg Work #3	4 x 10 times	4 x 15 times	4 x 20 times
Arm Work #5	4 x 10 times	4 x 15 times	4 x 20 times
Ab Work #4 & 5	4 x 10 times	4 x 15 times	4 x 20 times
Ball Work #1 & 4	4 x 10 times	4 x 15 times	4 x 20 times

DAY 4: SLEEP

Promise: *"And he cometh, and findeth them sleeping, and saith unto Peter, Simon, sleepest thou? couldest not thou watch one hour? Watch ye and pray, lest ye enter into temptation. The spirit truly is ready, but the flesh is weak. And again he went away, and prayed, and spake the same words. And when he returned, he found them asleep again, (for their eyes were heavy,) neither wist they what to answer him"* (Mark 14:37-40).

Practice: Waking early to seek the Lord is a reoccurring theme for many powerfully effective leaders in the Bible. Jesus rose early to pray (Mark 1:35). Joshua rose early to move forward in crossing the Jordan (Joshua 3:1). The landowner rose early to look for workers (Matthew 20:1). Job rose early to worship and offer sacrifices to the Lord (Job 1:5). Jesus had power, authority, and great discipline. After His death and burial, He rose again early on the third day. Joshua accomplished great feats in his flawless leadership following Moses. He obviously had no problem with sacrificing his sleep to gain a promised possession. The landowner was obviously a wealthy man. Perhaps the diligent workers arrived early. Then there is the faithful Job whose faithful practice of worship and sacrifice agitates satan himself. The comments made by the wicked one indicate that Job's entire life was protected by the fortress of God.

All of these men were prosperous and powerful. They also knew that there was immense power in rising early, often while it was yet night, to pray, praise, and worship the Lord. Is your schedule tight? Does it seem like you just cannot get a handle on your day? Are your losses greater than your wins throughout the day? Do you seem whipped when you go to bed and whipped when you wake up? Does it seem like your prayers are ignored? Perhaps you should consider the tactics that the aforementioned men of the Bible used.

When I was in the Amazon during my stay on the show, we took turns watching the fire and the camp throughout the night. We had to keep the fire going, for it was difficult to rekindle and necessary for sterilizing our water. It was also the job of the person watching to listen for wild animals and unusual sounds approaching the camp. I later learned that, in biblical times, the daytime hours were broken into four three-hour windows called "hours," and the nighttime hours were broken down into four three-hour windows called "watches." Prior to learning the power of finding intimacy with God during the forth watch, this was my time to exercise and study. More than any other time of the day, worship and study during the hours of 3 to 6 a.m. was beneficial and life-changing. I have gained great insight, wisdom, and revelation during the fourth watch. The ability to consistently do this is a show of great virtue: *"She riseth also while it is yet night, and giveth meat to her household, and a portion to her maidens"* (Proverbs 31:15). Is it possible that your breakthrough and blessing is floating around in the still of the early morning while most remain asleep, most phones are off, and stores are closed, along with eyes and mouths? I believe that during these hours, the air is clear and distractions are gone. Plan a day or two where you will subtract one hour from your sleep to sacrifice for praise, prayer, study, and exercise. There is power in sacrificing your sleep to tap into the power of the Most High God and the inner-strength that He has given you.

Prayer: Father God, I thank you for giving me, your beloved, sweet sleep. In the sweetness of the sleep you give me, I am refreshed for the challenges of a new day. Help me, oh Lord, to sacrifice a little sleep for the great benefits of beginning my day under the complete rule and plan of the Holy Spirit. I ask you even now, oh Lord, for the ear of the learned that I may hear and hearken unto your voice and know the path that I should take, day to day. I seek your face, oh Lord, for a change in my faith and a change in life. I am willing to do whatever it takes to move to the next level.

I am willing to enter my bed early so that I may exit my bed early and seek your face. I ask you to be my spiritual alarm speaking to my heart as I seek you early. I ask you even now, oh Lord, for courage, strength, structure, and discipline, that I might gain the same favor, insight, power, and prosperity of those in the Bible who rose early in the morning, making sleep the first of their sacrifices. Amen.

Psalm 139:1-10: *"O lord, thou hast searched me, and known me. Thou knowest my downsitting and mine uprising, thou understandest my thought afar off. Thou compassest my path and my lying down, and art acquainted with all my ways. For there is not a word in my tongue, but, lo, O LORD, thou knowest it altogether. Thou hast beset me behind and before, and laid thine hand upon me. Such knowledge is too wonderful for me; it is high, I cannot attain unto it. Whither shall I go from thy spirit? or whither shall I flee from thy presence? If I ascend up into heaven, thou art there: if I make my bed in hell, behold, thou art there. If I take the wings of the morning, and dwell in the uttermost parts of the sea; Even there shall thy hand lead me, and thy right hand shall hold me."*

Physical Activity:

1. Warm-up
2. Stretch
3. Workout Card: Day 4 – Workout Phase 4

EXERCISE: DAY 4	BEGINNER	MODERATE	ADVANCED
Cardio #4	4 x 25 non-stop	7 minutes	10 minutes
Leg Work #4	4 x 10 times	4 x 15 times	4 x 20 times
Arm Work #1 & 2	4 x 10 times	4 x 15 times	4 x 20 times
Ab Work #3 & 4	4 x 10 times	4 x 15 times	4 x 20 times
Ball Work #1 & 5	4 x 10 times	4 x 15 times	4 x 20 times

DAY 5: FASTING

Promise: *"Is not this the fast that I have chosen? to loose the bands of wickedness, to undo the heavy burdens, and to let the oppressed go free, and that ye break every yoke? Is it not to deal thy bread to the hungry, and that thou bring the poor that are cast out to thy house? when thou seest the naked, that thou cover him; and that thou hide not thyself from thine own flesh? Then shall thy light break forth as the morning, and thine health shall spring forth speedily: and thy righteousness shall go before thee; the glory of the LORD shall be thy rereward"* (Isaiah 58:6-8).

Practice: There are so many benefits to fasting and praying. Throughout the Bible, time after time, miracles were performed and spiritual growth was achieved through sincere fasting and praying. Here, in the book of Isaiah, fasting is described as a compilation of all the days we have covered thus far in this section of *The Fruit of Sacrifice*. A mere denial of eating, while considered fasting, is not what makes your light break forth, or what causes your health to spring forth speedily. It is a complete denial of all that pleases and comforts you. This is also indicated in the Spirit-led isolation of Jesus' forty day fast in the wilderness to be tempted by the devil. There is great purpose behind a true fast. A true fast is a self-inflicted form of ultimate discipline. When I dwelled on the jungle floor of the Amazon rainforest, I awoke every morning with the sole purposes of collecting and purifying water for the day. I also hoped, each day, to find food. There were no hair appointments, television shows scheduled, or trips to the convenience store. Surviving the day was my only work. When all was said and done, we needed to stay alive. To do that, our primary resource was food, second only to water.

If we can learn to deny *ourselves* food and water, the very things that keep us functioning and alive, then we will have very little difficulty conquering our bad habits and vices. The simple act of not eating can carry many motives other than that of spiritual significance and breakthrough. An individual who decides not to eat can be identified as having several eating disorders or using a very dangerous method to achieve a false sense of vanity. Let us really situate ourselves to activate the power and change that a true fast can bring about.

While there are many methods of fasting, the one I favor is supported by scientific evidence and is found in one of my most closely referenced nutritional books, *Prescription for Nutritional Healing* by Phyllis and James Balch. Many people take into consideration fasting for a certain number of hours or until a specified time of day. However, when Queen Esther realized Haman's plot to destroy her and her people, she called a three-day fast and gave specific instructions to her maidens and people not to eat or drink anything for three days and three nights (Esther 4:16). Not only did Esther maintain her royal position, her uncle was elevated, her people were spared, and her enemy Haman was destroyed, as were his sons. Fasting—while it is a great sacrifice in a world of donuts and coffee, shrimp and steak, cake and ice cream, just to name a few—is what pays the "light" bill in the life of a Christian.

Do you long for a major breakthrough? Are you looking to see the hand of God move in your home, on your job, or in your physical body? Have you tried half-hearted fasts only to find yourself irritable with a major headache? Take it seriously and do your research. Like anything else, the digestive system needs a break. Your body is designed to heal itself, but it is often preoccupied digesting heavy foods. Think about this: Take a big burger or steak, some French fries or a potato, and some vegetables or cheese sticks. You can gather these items literally or just as an image in your mind. Don't touch the food, just take a long look at it. Now everything you see on your mental or physical plate has to go into your body and be separated as either waste or nutrients. When it is a bunch of waste, your body has a very hard time processing the waste with little nutrients. If you have abused your digestive system by not keeping it clean and flowing with fresh fruits and vegetables, it will store waste more frequently and digest food more slowly. Give your digestive system a break by eating only foods power-packed with nutrients that it can use to heal your body. You are worth it. Add prayer, meditation, and an hourly intake of God's Word to your fast and you will see your health spring forth speedily and long-awaited miracles will begin to take place. Remember: All of these changes begin with you!

Prayer: Father God, I thank you that I have food to eat. Help me to understand the importance of what I eat and how it affects my body. Father God, I pray for the temperance and self-discipline to fast not only from food, but from anything that I really enjoy. Lord, during my time of fasting, I offer my all to you so that I will need and desire only you. Help me to gain full insight and wisdom about the powerful physical and spiritual benefits of true fasting.

Your Word teaches me that I should not live by bread alone, but by your Word. Help me, oh Lord, to make my first and last meal of the day be a full course of your Word. Lord, I dedicate one day of my week to fasting and praying about the things that are on my heart and the situations that seem like they are out of control in my life. I trust your Holy Spirit to set a watch at my mouth from this day forth to guard what goes in and what comes out.

Father, I pray that I may walk a fasting life layered with temperance and self-restraint, eradicating the urge to *indulge* myself in anything other than prayer, praise, and your Word. Help me to say *no* to myself more often than I say *yes*. Give me the sound realization that I control my appetite, eating habits, and actions. They do not control me. Make me over, Lord. I can do this and all things through Christ who strengthens me. Amen.

Psalm 42: 1-4: *"As the hart panteth after the water brooks, so panteth my soul after thee, O God. My soul thirsteth for God, for the living God: when shall I come and appear before God? My tears have been my meat day and night, while they continually say unto me, Where is thy God? When I remember these things, I pour out my soul in me: for I had gone with the multitude, I went with them to the house of God, with the voice of joy and praise, with a multitude that kept holyday."*

Physical Activity:
1. Warm-up
2. Stretch
3. Workout Card: Day 5 – Workout Phase 4

EXERCISE: DAY 5	BEGINNER	MODERATE	ADVANCED
Cardio	#1 x 17 minutes	#2 x 12 minutes	#3 x 9 minutes
Leg Work #5	4 x 10 times	4 x 15 times	4 x 20 times
Arm Work #3 & 4	4 x 10 times	4 x 15 times	4 x 20 times
Ab Work #5 & 1	4 x 10 times	4 x 15 times	4 x 20 times
Ball Work #1 & 2	4 x 10 times	4 x 15 times	4 x 20 times

DAY 6: FORGIVENESS

Promise: *"Then came Peter to him, and said, Lord, how oft shall my brother sin against me, and I forgive him? till seven times? Jesus saith unto him, I say not unto thee, Until seven times: but, Until seventy times seven"* (Matthew 18:21-22).

Practice: Forgiveness is one of the most powerful weapons of warfare a person may acquire. Notice that I said *acquire*, not *have*. Forgiveness is a costly choice that, until activated, leaves the one lacking it full of bitterness and anger. In many of my small group counseling sessions filled with children dealing with divorce, we spend over three quarters of our time together on forgiveness. Until they forgive themselves and then those whom they feel have offended them, anything else we address is fruitless. I can see the pain and disappointment in their eyes as they move from blaming their teachers, their friends, the cat, the dog, and even themselves. They blame everyone and everything to avoid the truth of simply being angry with their parents' decision of divorce. Often, they blame the parent who seems to have caused the inconvenient disruption in their seemingly happy home without being at all interested in the reasoning behind that parent's action. All they know is that they have been inconveniently disrupted, and they could care less about why it actually happened.

Without intervention, these children turn into adults who feel justified in being bitter and unforgiving. Forgiveness, though expressed outwardly, is an inward remedy for the soul of the one expressing it. Forgiveness allows a person to move on in freedom, opportunity, love, growth, and fellowship. Some people, like the children in my group, have blamed someone for something in their past that did not turn out the way they wanted or expected it to. Some of these people may have experienced disappointment, rejection, or ultimate betrayal. However long the list may be, letting go of it is key to moving forward, growing and becoming prepared for a higher calling.

In Psalms 90:12, Moses prays that God will teach us to number our days that we may apply our hearts unto wisdom. Each day that passes without forgiveness is lost and may be considered a compiled repetition of days from the past filled with the situation that caused the hurt. More intensely, there are those who literally have issues of forgiveness with God himself. God is God, and His track record, while not accommodating all of our desires and quirks, and sometimes not even taking into consideration our finite understanding, is indeed flawless. Yet, because of some detrimental, unexplainable, seemingly irrational thing that God has *allowed* to happen to us as human beings, some people harbor bitterness and a secretly justified resentment toward God's decision for our lives.

Much like the children in my counseling group, many people, especially believers who consider themselves immune to tragedy and disappointment, simply cannot forgive God for seemingly unnecessary pain. Jesus prayed as the true and only begotten Son of God in the Garden of Gethsemane that the cup of separation through crucifixion would pass; but His request was denied. In His final breaths on the cross, Jesus, while asking for the forgiveness of those persecuting Him, questioned the one in whom He placed His trust and confidence. Christ, in His flawless walk of existence in human flesh, simultaneously forgave His trespassers while questioning the Father's decision of temporary divorce.

"And at the ninth hour Jesus cried with a loud voice, saying, Eloi, Eloi, lama sabachthani? which is, being interpreted, 'My God, my God, why hast thou forsaken me?'" (Mark 15:34).

Where do you stand with walking in a spirit of forgiveness? The Bible instructs us to be angry but sin not and to never let the sun go down on our anger or wrath, but I am not talking about an episode or argument. I am talking about that thing that you may have deep down in your soul that you have never let go of and until today you have never intended to let go of. It grabbed hold of you and it has altered your personality and, therefore, the genuine interaction you should have with others. Let it go, as Jesus did at the hands of His haters. Take it to God in prayer, daily, until you know that you know that you know that you have let that *thing* go. Then go to your brother and both forgive and ask for forgiveness.

It works. It releases you first, and then it releases the person who is probably hindered by knowing your feelings toward him or her. Even if you have issues with what God has allowed to happen in your life, tell Him about them. Cry with a loud voice and express your pain to God in the name of Jesus Christ. God cares so much about your disappointments that He manifested himself in the flesh of Jesus Christ to prove to you that He loves you. He cares about your suffering and feels your pain. *"For we have not an high priest which cannot be touched with the feeling of our infirmities; but was in all points tempted like as we are, yet without sin"* (Hebrews 4:15). Forgiveness is not only a sacrifice, it is a daily choice that matures us and truly reveals to us who God is and the role He has for us to enact here on Earth. Choose forgiveness today and feel the release in your heart while watching a mighty move of God in your life.

Prayer: Father God, grant us the serenity to accept the things from the past, present, and future that we can never change with all of our might and effective prayer. Dear Lord, grant us divine courage in identifying and acting upon those things within ourselves that we can change through the Lord Jesus Christ. Lord, grant us the wisdom to know the difference between the things and the people of the past that we cannot change and the daily choices we can make that will impact our futures from this day forward.

Father God, I choose to live, move, and breathe in complete forgiveness. Purge me with hyssop that I might be clean. Wash me that I might be whiter than snow. Create in me a clean heart, a clean mind, and renew a right spirit of forgiveness within me. In my family, oh God, I ask for reconciliation to spring forth where relationships have been severed due to occurrences in my past. I choose forgiveness, Father, and I accept your forgiveness even when I can find none among my family or fellow man. I accept your forgiveness, and I ask for the insight and humility to walk with a heart so saturated with the blood of Jesus Christ that hatred, bitterness, anger, wrath, or revenge never take root again. I am a forgiving person, and I will never be set back again by being unforgiving. I am willing to sacrifice my pride and the possibility of being hurt again for the freedom of forgiveness.

I trust you, Lord, and I trust in the plans that you have for my life. Search my heart, oh Lord, for secret faults and underlying issues that I may not know about. Reveal to me the places of my heart so dark, deep, and suppressed that I may not even know they are there. You know all things, Father. There is nothing hidden from you. You know all about me, and I love you for that. I am willing, ready, and able, through Christ Jesus, to forgive those who have harmed me, for they did not know what they were doing to me in fulfillment of their own desires. Lord God, even you say in your Word that you forgive us not for us but for your own sake: "I, even I, am he that blotteth out thy transgressions for mine own sake, and will not remember thy sins" (Isaiah 43:25). I, too, for my own sake, choose to forgive and to move on in the name of Jesus Christ. Hallelujah! Oh Glory! Hallelujah! Amen!

Psalm 51:17-19: *"The sacrifices of God are a broken spirit: a broken and a contrite heart, O God, thou wilt not despise. Do good in thy good pleasure unto Zion: build thou the walls of Jerusalem. Then shalt thou be pleased with the sacrifices of righteousness, with burnt offering and whole burnt offering: then shall they offer bullocks upon thine altar."*

Physical Activity:
1. Warm-up
2. Stretch
3. Workout Card: Day 6 – Workout Phase 4

EXERCISE: DAY 6	BEGINNER	MODERATE	ADVANCED
Cardio #4	25 non-stop	7 minutes	10 minutes
Cardio #5	10 minutes	15 minutes	20 minutes
Leg Work #1	4 x 10 times	4 x 15 times	4 x 20 times
Arm Work #5	4 x 10 times	4 x 15 times	4 x 20 times
Ab Work #1 & 2	4 x 10 times	4 x 15 times	4 x 20 times
Ball Work #1 & 3	4 x 10 times	4 x 15 times	4 x 20 times

DAY 7: THE FLESH

Promise: *"I beseech you therefore, brethren, by the mercies of God, that ye present your bodies a living sacrifice, holy, acceptable unto God, which is your reasonable service. And be not conformed to this world: but be ye transformed by the renewing of your mind, that ye may prove what is that good, and acceptable, and perfect, will of God"* (Romans 12:1-2).

Practice: How does one present her body of flesh as a living, breathing sacrifice to God, and why is it considered a sacrifice? The Word of God constantly reminds us of the lack of good things in our flesh. If the flesh is not crucified or brought under subjection daily, it will begin to rule us and give into our human nature of sin. However, when we present our bodies to God, we bring them under subjection of the Holy Spirit who governs our steps and guides our decision-making. Physical subjection to the service and will of God is a precious gift to God. When you give your body over to Christ through the Holy Spirit of Truth, you become the eyes, arms, feet, and mind of God:

"For though we walk in the flesh, we do not war after the flesh. (For the weapons of our warfare are not carnal but mighty through God to the pulling down of strong holds;) Casting down imaginations, and every high thing that exalteth itself against the knowledge of God, and bringing into captivity every thought to the obedience of Christ; And having in a readiness to revenge all disobedience, when your obedience is fulfilled" (2 Corinthians 10:3-6).

This is a foundational Scripture, as it pertains to our walk in the flesh. The true warfare, while manifested in the flesh, is derived through our spiritual and mental foundations. This is why the foundation of this book addresses the balance of the whole woman or man in moving forward physically. Again, the flesh is subjected to a made-up mind and a spirit that has sold out to God. However, with all of this knowledge, we are still moved by a wall of vulnerable flesh that requires daily submission to Christ and lots of discipline and self-control. This, then, supports the fact that the spirit is willing while the flesh is weak. Paul clearly states that he is clear on what to do, yet that is not what he does, and what he does he knows he should not do. Paul also states that there is a thorn in his flesh, a messenger of satan who was sent to buffet him, and he went before God about this thorn three times. Paul concludes that the thorn is there to keep him humble before God so that he will not begin to exalt himself. God gave Paul an imperfection so that Paul would know that God's grace was sufficient and that, even in the weak points of Paul's flesh, God would be made strong.

Hallelujah! That is not an excuse for us to allow our bodies to run rampant in fulfilling their every desire, but we are to realize that we need God each and every day of our lives to stay well spiritually and physically, not just twenty-eight days in a devotional. Even if you've failed to complete other fitness programs, it's OK. Ask God to help you complete *this program* and make daily devotion and fitness a regular part of your life.

This means devoting our lives and bodies to Christ through our everyday actions of sacrifice and love. We must see Christ in our mirrors. We must see Christ in our jeans and shirts. We must see Jesus in our skirts and dresses. This is the only way we will ever find any perfection or goodness in our flesh. Jesus gave the perfect example of how to sacrifice the flesh back to God. We were crucified with Christ on that cross. This is a conviction through faith. This is where our Savior originally crucified our flesh. Now it is our time for us to walk in that level of authority over the wiles, desires, and deep cravings of the flesh. God will perfect that which pertains to you, and he will not forsake the work of His hands. (See Psalms 138:8.)

You can have victory through Christ even in your flesh, just as He did. Greater is he who is in Christ Jesus than he who is in the world. Hallelujah! That is great news! Today, give your body to Christ. Allow God to take control. In this gift to God, you will find a new and improved you. You will experience the manifestation of God's perfection in your flesh. Moses' relationship with God kept his eyes from growing dim and his body from aging. (See Deuteronomy 34:7.) I believe that God is faithful. I know that when I sacrificed my body to God during my junior year in college, in obedience to having my son as opposed to aborting him, God set my body on a path of preservation that is far better than my pre-childbirth physical state was. I am in much better spiritual, emotional, and physical condition than I was fifteen years ago as a college basketball player.

Since then, I have learned to survive the fitness game and still play an impressive full-speed, full-court basketball game. I do not have stretch marks on my abdomen. From looking at me, it is hard to determine that I am the mother of a 291-pound offensive lineman. I am a very proud mother, only by the grace of God.

What is God calling you to do with your body? Does He want to restore your waistline? Does He want to bring forth children in your life through your womb or adoption, but you have *selfishly* put Him on hold? What is going on with your body? Where does God need your hands to be? Who needs to see God's smile or hear His voice through you? Where are you with your body and where is God trying to take you? Completely surrender to Him. Just as He gave you your body, He has a great and mighty plan for it. (See Jeremiah 33:3.) Submit your body to God today as a living, breathing sacrifice, and reap the fruit of long life, health, prosperity, and peace in God.

Prayer: Lord Jesus, I thank you for giving me an example of perfect obedience and sacrifice through your walk here on earth in the flesh. Teach me to die to my fleshly desires and motives daily that I might do the will of the Father and fulfill my destiny. Father God, I present my body to you as a living sacrifice today and for the rest of my stay here on Earth. After preparing me, I ask, Father God, that you use me to perform your works and will daily. Let your will be done through me here on Earth as it is being done in Heaven. Take me and make me, hold me and mold me, choose me and use me for all that you created me to be and to do. I am willing and I am ready, Father, to make the necessary sacrifices to go to the next level. I am ready to live by the faith that the *just* in Christ live by. I am ready and willing to live my life by faith and not by sight, increasing my faith through the hearing, studying, and obeying of your Word. I am a sinner saved by your grace, God, and I know that your grace is sufficient to deliver me and to provide me a way of escape from all of the snares and shortcomings I make. Be glorified in my flesh and my body.

Lord, I know that faith without works is dead, and, as I work toward walking in a physical way that is not only pleasing to you but gives you great glory, please honor and bless my efforts and make them fruitful.

I trust you with everything.

I am your creation, and you are the author and finisher of my faith. Complete this work that you began in me while I am still surviving the game of life. Once I have played my last quarter here on Earth, let your greeting be for me, with open arms: "Well done, my good and faithful servant, well done." Amen. Amen. Amen.

Psalm 63:1: *"O God, thou art my God; early will I seek thee: my soul thirsteth for thee, my flesh longeth for thee in a dry and thirsty land, where no water is."*

Physical Activity:
1. Warm-up
2. Stretch
3. Workout Card: Day 7 – Workout Phase 4

EXERCISE: DAY 7	BEGINNER	MODERATE	ADVANCED
	REST	REST	REST

Day 7—Remember the Sabbath day and to keep it holy, and God will remember you. God rested on the seventh day, and so should you!

Descriptions and Instructions for Core Exercises

(Please watch the DVD for demonstrations.)

Core 1: Cardio Exercises

The **Core Cardio Exercises** are designed to condition your lungs and heart while helping your body burn fat:

Walking, Running, and Jogging:

These should be done in very comfortable shoes and light clothing. When covering distances over one mile, or when in motion longer than fifteen minutes, you must take your water along with you. These Core Cardio Exercises may be monitored by distance or, better yet, by time. If you do not have access to a track to monitor laps, use landmarks like a store, a house, or a parking lot. Take into consideration both climate and time of day when you work out outside. If the day is hot, then the early mornings or late evenings may be the best time for you. However, if you choose to walk, run, or jog during sundown hours, it is imperative that you do the following:

A) Make yourself visible through the use of reflectors or reflective clothing.

B) If you have to go alone, always tell someone where you are going and when you expect to be back.

C) Always carry your cell phone and a form of identification.

1. Fitness Walking: 110 yards at 1 minute 15 seconds or less is considered fitness walking at a moderate pace. A mile completed in 20 minutes is a moderate pace. There is a difference between Fitness Walking and a daily stroll through the park. Fitness walking is taking extended strides while engaging the arms, abdominal region, and your cardio-respiratory system. Next to pool aerobics, this is the best and most effective exercise for the beginner.

2. Jogging: 110 yards at 45 seconds or less is considered jogging. A mile completed in 12 minutes is a slow jog. This is the next step after the highest level of Fitness Walking. Jogging is Fitness Walking adding the ballistic movements of the knees and feet in forward motion. It can be accomplished in a very low form. Your challenge can either be the distance you run or a constant decrease in the time you run a consistent distance. For example, if it takes you 12 minutes to run around your neighborhood in your Pre-program, you should be down to at least 10 minutes in your Post-program. That is a decrease of about 30 seconds per week, 7-10 seconds per workout.

3. Running: 110 yards at 26 seconds or less is considered running. A mile run in 7 minutes is considered a slow run. This exercise would best suit those who are already physically active and would like to break a plateau, add structure to an existing routine, or learn how to move from walking or jogging to running.

4. Jumping Rope. This cardio exercise is all-inclusive in that it gives the body a full workout that involves a combination of toning and cardio. To be effective at jumping rope, a bare floor or other non-impaired surface is best. Also, baggy, cumbersome clothing may impede the rhythm of your jump or the flow of your rope. The correct jump rope for you is one long enough to reach from armpit to armpit, passing under both feet.

For beginners, try counting the highest number of times you can turn and clear the rope without error. The best 3 out of 5 attempts should be used to gauge your Pre-program max. After being able to jump over 100 times successfully, you are ready to gauge your roping by timed intervals. *Jumping rope for 2 minutes and 30 seconds without stop is moderate jumping.*

5. Cardio dance. This exercise is very fun and should be done based on durations of no less than 3 minutes. Cardio dance in a constant movement that includes using your arm and legs. You can tap your feet side to side. You can tap your heels forward. You can march forward and backwards. Just keep everything in motion until the end of your favorite song. Your level of intensity should be so that you have to catch your breath at the end of the song along with possible light perspiration. *One song is a warm-up—3 to 5 minutes. Two additional songs are considered slow cardio—6 to 10 minutes.*

Core 2: Leg Work Exercises

The **Core Leg Work Exercises** are designed to firm and tone your legs, hips, and glutes.

Lunges and Squats:

These may be performed either walking or standing in place. *They are not recommended for those with knee problems.* Another key point about lunges is that they are designed to intensely engage the quadriceps and hamstrings while placing minimum work on the knees. Because the knees have tendons and ligaments that do not "immediately" express the same work load burden as muscles, some participants shift all of their body weight to the knees. It simply "feels" easier. The long-term effect, however, is detrimental. Be sure that you always keep your knees behind your ankles. If your knees protrude in front of your ankles, attempt to correct your posture by stepping forward with the knee above the ankle, not in front of it, while engaging and feeling the workload in your quadriceps (thighs). If you cannot correct your posture, then move on to a less complex exercise in Core 2. Squats are similar to lunges, but we are going to use the chair to insure that they are performed correctly. Sitting slightly on the edge of your chair, you should look down to see that your knees are lined up with your ankles or behind them, never forward of your ankles. Without using your hands, stand all the way up, squeezing your behind with the stand and sitting back down before releasing the squeeze.

This may be performed for your inner thighs by pointing your toes out to the sides and still keeping your knees behind your ankles.

1. Lunges: For the beginner, stand straight up with both legs together and with your hands on your hips. Step forward as far as you can, slightly bending your knee without extending it past your ankle. Bring your leg back into place with the other and continue alternating this sequence to acquire your Pre-program maximum. *Intermediate exercisers should be able to complete no less than 1 set of 15 repetitions on each leg. A lower and deeper lunge should be developed over the next four weeks.*

2. Squats: Using the chair for accuracy, an intermediate exerciser should be able to perform no less than 1 set of 25 repetitions. Speed can be used as a method of simultaneously adding cardio to this toner.

Glute Squeezes and Lying Side Leg Lifts:

These exercises are designed to target saddle bags (puddles of fat on the hips) and lift the rear end, which is also termed the gluteus muscle.

3. Glute Squeezes: Using your mat, lie flat on your back with your knees bent, arms parallel to your body, and palms flat on floor. Lift your hips off of your mat as high as you can. Hold this position for one full second and return to a fully relaxed position. *One set of 20 repetitions is moderate for gluteus squeezes.*

4. Lying Side Leg Lifts: Using your mat, lie on your side supporting your head with your arm. With the leg closest to the floor bent, lift the top leg as high as you can and bring it back down to the opposite leg. For beginners or those who have problems getting off of the floor, follow the same technique standing assisted by the back of the chair with the seat facing away from your body. Gradually increase the height of your leg lift with each workout. *One set of 20 repetitions is moderate for lying side leg lifts.*

5. Basic Step Up: This is one of my favorite exercises for burning calories, fat, and toning the legs. This exercise may be cautiously implemented anywhere that there are steps with a railing. You may also purchase a step with various height ranges to adjust with the growth of your exercise program. When you step up, you should feel a comfortable, natural burn from the workload, not a struggle or strain. If you feel a struggle or strain, adjust your step to a lower height until a level of natural comfort is reached. Step up and then down on the step using the same leg for 15 repetitions; or alternate legs for each step up.

This exercise may be used with your 32 count music on the same basis as the cardio dance explained later on. *One set of 15 Basic Step Ups per leg is considered moderate step. Adjustment of height and an increase of repetitions are recommended to achieve a continued exercise benefit.*

Core 3: Arm Work Exercises

The **Core Arm Work Exercises** are designed to tone the arms. *"She girdeth her loins with strength and strengtheneth her arms"* (Proverbs 31: 17).

1. Biceps and 2. Triceps:

Begin with as little as one pound hand weights. If hand weights are not available, then water bottles, canned goods, or even a pair of running shoes may be used for resistance. To avoid bulking and building muscle, it is recommended that 10 pounds be the maximum weight used. To obtain optimal results in toning and leaning, increase the number of repetitions used. **Bicep** muscles are located on the **front side** of each arm midway between the shoulders and the elbows. **Triceps** are muscles located on the **back side** of each arm midway between the shoulders and the elbows. Bicep curls should begin by grasping your weights or weighted objects with the palms facing forward or up.

Beginning with arms fully extended down, gently lift your forearms from the upper thigh area to the shoulders and back down. This counts as one repetition. Begin working triceps by standing straight up and then leaning, slightly forward, with weights or weighted objects at your sides. Curl the weights up to your shoulders as you would for the bicep curl, keeping the elbows bent and high. Fully extend the forearm only behind you. Do not rotate your shoulders, only the forearm bending at the elbow. Curl back up to your shoulders. This counts as one repetition.

Bicep curls may be done for a specified duration or for a specific count. You may implement hand weights three pounds or less with cardio dance, walking, jogging, lunges, squats, or step ups. Keeping small hand weights in your hands always adds more toning to your arms and intensity to your workout.

Biceps: 1 set of 15 repetitions is a moderate workload.
Triceps: 1 set of 15 repetitions is a moderate workload.

3. Shoulder Presses: The weight recommendations and strategy are the same for the entire area core sections. Shoulder presses help with balance and posture. With shoulder presses, the upper back is also toned. These next two arm exercises may seem more difficult because you rarely lift your arms above your head. These muscles are rarely used throughout the day, and, if they are used, it is not with weights for an excess of 15 repetitions. Standing straight up, hold the weights in your hands. Lift your arms bending at the elbow so that your fists are parallel with your ears only being separated by the upper arm area. Fully extend both arms above your head until the weights touch. Bring your arms back to the starting position, making your elbows even with your shoulders and your fists even with your ears.

These lifts may be done for a specified duration or a specific count. *One set of 15 repetitions count as a moderate workload.*

4. Deltoid Lifts: Deltoid lifts focuses on the posterior shoulders. Your deltoid muscles are located from the top of your shoulders down to the first third of your arm. To effectively perform the deltoid exercise, grasp your weights or weighted objects with your arms bent at the elbows. Keep your elbows close to your body. Your forearm should be positioned so that your hands and elbows are parallel. Without moving your forearm, lift them up and out to the side until they are slightly higher than the shoulders. Return to your original position. This counts as one repetition.

These lifts may be done for a specified duration or a specific count. *One set of 15 repetitions count as a moderate workload.*

5. Chest Press: The chest press primarily focuses on the lifting and toning of the bust area. If you have problems with oversized breasts or sagging, this exercise can help with both. Chest presses may be performed lying on the mat or standing. With your forearms facing straight up with your elbows away from your body, grasp your weights. Slowly bring your elbows in toward your body, keeping the forearms straight up. Return to your original position. This counts as one repetition.

These presses may be done for a specified duration or a specific count. *One set of 15 repetitions counts as a moderate workload.*

Core 4: Abdominal Work Exercises

The **Core Abdominal Work Exercises** are designed to uniquely trim fat around the entire upper body region, also termed the lumbar system.

1. Basic Sit-Ups and 2. Crunches:

1. Basic Sit-Ups: Basic sit-ups are an age-old traditional workout that tones the middle abdominals and the back muscles. If you need support for your feet, you can have someone help you, or you can place your feet midway beneath a sofa, chair, couch, or bed. Lying flat on your mat with your knees bent and your feet flat, support your head with your hands and lift your torso as high as you can. Gently return to your original position.

Because your neck and back muscles are involved, take care to perform each repetition slowly and carefully. This exercise may be combined with crunches in 50/50 intervals. For example, 10 sit-ups followed by 10 crunches with a 15-second break. *10 sit-ups is a moderate level workload. One set of 20 crunches is considered a moderate workload.*

2. Crunches: Crunches are performed in the same position. To perform an accurate crunch, keep your elbows pointed away from your body, parallel with your ears. Come up to the highest point of resistance without lifting completely off of the floor. Your shoulders through the mid-back area should leave the floor.

Both sit-ups and crunches may be shifted to either side dominantly to emphasize strategic work loads on the right and left side obliques. To work the left side, lift the right arm, bended elbow, with right hand behind your head over to the left, and vice versa for your right side.

3. Curl Crunch: You may have never heard of an abdominal exercise termed Curl Crunch because this is one of my personal techniques and a favorite for engaging the upper, lower, and middle abdominals in one smooth, fluid motion. Rest flat on your back in the same position as described for the sit-ups and the crunches. Lying face-up, with your hands and legs fully extended, bring your knees and your arms together and squeeze your body into a ball. Return to your original position. You can either fully extend your body or return to the sit-up crunch position with your knees bent. This counts as 1 repetition. *One set of 15 Curl Crunches is a moderate workload.*

4. Hip Lifts: Lying flat on your back in the same position as described for the sit-ups and the crunches in 4.1-2, lift your legs into the air as high as you can, attempting to lift your hips off of the floor. To ensure secure balance for your back, you can place your hands or a towel at the middle of your back. This would be the mid-area between your waist and back. Most people do not need this support, but, if you do, place a towel or your hands behind you to fill the gap between the floor and your back.

This exercise may be performed by pushing your feet straight into the air as if your hands were tied and you were trying to kick the ceiling to get out. *15 consecutive lifts at this level are considered advanced.*

This exercise for beginners is performed in the same position with the same technique, but the knees are bent when up and bent when moving down, allowing the toes to tap the floor. *10 consecutive lifts is a beginner workload.*

5. Lying Cycle Peddles: This exercise is good for strengthening and toning the lower abdominals. Lying Cycle Peddles are strategic in targeting the "pudgy area" below the navel. Lying flat on your back, in the same position as described for the sit-ups and the crunches in 4.1-2, lift your knees above your waist with your feet slightly higher than your knees. Keep one knee up throughout the rotation while fully extending the other and lowering it to the floor. This exercise should be performed in an alternating pattern. For beginners, follow the same position and sequence, keeping the knee bent on the leg that goes to the floor, and alternating. *10 Lying Cycle Peddles on each leg at the advanced level is a moderate workload.*

Core 5: Ball Work Exercises

The **Core Ball Work Exercises** are designed to add variety and deliver deep, vigorous, and intense work to the abdominal region.

Basic Crunch, Full Fallback Sit-up, and Pelvic Tilts:

These exercises are performed using the fitness ball. Fitness balls range in size from 55cm to 75cm. If you are not sure which size is best for you, stick with the 55cm ball. It is better that your ball be too small than too large. When the ball is too large, balancing and control issues may occur. Persons 5'5 and under should use the 55cm ball. Persons between 5'6 and 6' should be able to comfortably use a 65cm ball. Persons over 6' should use the 75cm ball. Simply using the ball as a seat while on the telephone or while watching television, engages the lower abdominals. The ball keeps you off of the floor while fully conforming to fit every crevice of your body, leaving virtually no gaps. When you position yourself correctly, it feels like you are floating on air.

Learn to like your ball. It may seem awkward or cumbersome sitting on the ball at first, sort of like you might fall. Keeping your feet firmly planted on the floor provides great support for balance and control. Next, try to lie back on the ball like it is a bean bag chair. When lying back, keep your arms out to the side or above your head so that your arm may be able to touch the floor. This position is much like lying on the floor fully stretched out.

1. Basic Crunches on the ball are performed using the same techniques described in 4-2. The ball should cover the lower part of your back while your feet hold the base and your arms support your head. Lift up and down, engaging the middle and upper abdominals. This counts as one repetition. *One set of 20 Basic Crunches on the ball is a moderate workload.*

2. Full Fallback Sit-Ups are performed sitting on the front end of the ball in a slope position. Your feet should be spread wide and the upper part of your back should not make contact with the ball until you fall back and try to touch the floor behind you. You will come all the way up, reaching your elbows to your knees, then falling back to the original position. This counts as one repetition. *One set of 10 Full Fallback Sit-ups on the ball is a moderate workload.*

3. Pelvic Tilts are designed to "get rid of the gut." There is usually a significant pooling of fat in the outer pelvic area of the stomach. This usually occurs because this area of the stomach is rarely engaged directly in physical activities that combat fat. This method is called "spot" training. This means that we are targeting a specific trouble spot to get rid of fat and tone that area. *One set of 20 Pelvic Tilts on the ball is a moderate workload.*

Sitting with your back fully aligned with the ball and your rear end just above the floor, lift and curl your hips back toward your body. To engage your upper abs you can simultaneously bring your shoulder down while tilting the pelvic area. This exercise differs in intensity from "Pelvic Thrusts." Lifting and tilting the hips back toward the body alone or combined with the shoulders counts as 1 repetition.

4. Back Toner: This exercise is designed to reduce the fat that spills out of your bra, and it melts away back rolls that are easily seen through fitted clothes. The Back Toner is performed lying face forward on your ball, preferably with your knees bent and your feet against the wall or couch. Your hands and arms now provide the base support for your balance. With arms folded against your chest, lift your torso back toward your feet or the wall. Return back to a relaxed lying position. This counts as one repetition. *One set of 10 Back Toners on the ball is a moderate workload.*

In performing the **Advanced Back Toner,** lay flat across the ball with your legs out and supported by your arms. You should look like you are doing a full pushup with the ball beneath your stomach and waist. This exercise may be performed with or without weights. In the pushup position, lift each arm, bending at the elbow and pulling in a circular motion toward the opposite arm. The elbows should seem to target the center of your back. The right and left arms should be alternated respectively. *One set of 10 Advanced Back Toners on the ball is a moderate workload.*

5. Oblique Toner: This exercise is designed to define the upper oblique muscles. This is the area from beneath the arm pits to the waistline. Some people call these rolls of fat "Love Handles." Now that you are familiar and comfortable with lying forward and back on your ball, it is time to lie on your side using the ball. Cup the ball beneath your arm pit and waist. Leave the bottom leg straight while crossing it with the top leg bent and with a foot on the floor. This means that if you are lying on your right side, you should be supported by your right arm and a straightened right leg. Your balance will come from the right arm and left leg crossed over right with a foot on the floor. In your left hand, take a weight and push it to the floor. This is your "down position." Pull the same weight up and back until your elbow touches the ball. If you have a low range of motion or shortened arms, you may not be able to touch the ball behind you with your elbow. In this case, just pull as far as you can. Returning the weight to the floor with an extended elbow counts as one repetition. This should be repeated one side at a time. *1 set of 15 with or without weight provides a moderate workload.*

Acknowledgments

The opportunity that led to my becoming a first-time author was birthed from a real life tale of a young girl turned Amazon Queen who made it through life's challenges on a fuel known to the fittest as *survival*. Along the way, there were a brave few who saw the glimpses of the diamond within the rough, and through their individual thrust and blows this little girl has been hurled into the destiny of authoring *Surviving the Fitness Game*.

My love and appreciation to my son Dontre. You are my true motivation and constant reminder of how much God really wants the absolute best for us. Thank you for your patience, wisdom, obedience, and support. I love you.

I would like to thank my sister Nancy for her faithfulness to our family legacy of prayer, keeping the prophetic words of our mother above ground and filled with life, and taking a faith walk that rewarded her with a new lease on life. Thank you for being a midwife to the birthing of this project. I thank my brother David and sister (in-law) Marian Ward for your constant support. Thank you to my sister Pheba (Dee) for driving from Atlanta to Orangeburg to get me to the Amazon without delay. Thank you to my sister Gwendolyn, you have been so strong for so long. With joy we celebrate the birth of your first grandchild, my grand niece, Cherish Mariah Jackson, during this project. To my oldest sister Louise, thank you for your constant prayers.

Thank you to Marcellus Miller for encouraging and watering all of my visions with your God Factor principles. Yolander Lee Williams, I love you and thank God for your friendship. Thank you, Sylvester, for all that you do.

Thank you to Pat Robertson, Ivorie Anthony, and the rest of the 700 Club members and staff for you constant prayers and support.

Thank you to everyone at Bridge-Logos. Your expertise, professionalism, and prayers greatly added to my experience as a first-time author.

I would like to thank all of my students from South Carolina State University and Lexington School District #4. It has been a pleasure sharing faith and fitness with you.

Ms. Sarah Washington-Favors, Dr. Jessie & Shirley Kinard, Dr. Kenneth Mosely, Coach Willie Jeffries, Mrs. Geraldine Goodwin Outlaw, Dr. Howard Hill, Coach Kirk Collier, Dr. Willie B. Owens, and Barron Driskell: thanks so much for your encouragement and support during my wonder years.

To the Jamison sisters, I love you dearly and you are a treasure to my soul.

Thanks to the great folks of Dekalb County Georgia for being community oriented and fitness friendly.

This book is dedicated to our loving mother Dorothy Vassell, who prophesied that I would author many books in a season that I did not think it possible. Oh great and mighty woman of God, proclaiming His excellent greatness and high praises often in the midst of adversity. Mother, I thank you for leaving a priceless legacy worth its weight in gold of faith, praise, and worship of the Most High El-Elyon God. Thank you so much for demanding excellence, challenging our potential, and instilling in all of us the rare qualities of integrity and Godly character. God in charge, God in control! Hallelujah! The Lord shall increase us more and more, me and all of your children. Psalm 115:14.